Rehabilitation Outcome Measures

Commissioning Editor: Rita Demetriou-Swanwick
Development Editor: Veronika Watkins
Project Manager: Jess Thompson
Designer: Kirsteen Wright
Illustration Manager: Gillian Richards
Illustrator: Chartwell Illustrators

Rehabilitation Outcome Measures

By
Emma K. Stokes
Senior Lecturer, Department of Physiotherapy, School of Medicine,
Trinity College, Dublin

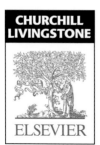

Edinburgh London New York Oxford Philadelphia St Louis Sydney Toronto 2011

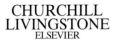

CHURCHILL
LIVINGSTONE
ELSEVIER

ISBN 978-0-443-06915-4

British Library Cataloguing in Publication Data
A catalogue record for this book is available from the British Library

Library of Congress Cataloging in Publication Data
A catalog record for this book is available from the Library of Congress

Printed in China

Contents

Dedication

This book is dedicated to my parents, John and Margaret Stokes, whose ever present love, support, encouragement and belief in all my endeavours is the constant that brings them to fruition.

Acknowledgements

A book written by one author is rarely the work of just that one individual.

I have drawn inspiration from the books of Professor Ian McDowell and Dr Claire Newell, and Professor Elspeth Finch and colleagues. I gratefully acknowledge the permissions received from authors and publishers to adapt and reproduce the work of others, especially in Section 4 of this book which brings all the outcome measures to the readers. I wish to thank Ralph Hammond and Dr Sarah Mitchell whose enthusiasm for this project gave me the impetus to forge ahead and to Professor Des O'Neill who supervised the initial work which resulted in the first two sections of the book.

I am very grateful to Deirdre Lynch and Jenny Stokes whose valuable administrative assistance enabled the final stages of the compilation of the book to be achieved and to Veronika Watkins, Development Editor at Elsevier for her patience and guidance in the preparation of the manuscript.

I wish also to acknowledge my friends Professor John O'Hagan and Professor Linda Doyle whose ongoing interest in and questioning about this project and my PhD, which formed the basis for my interest in this field, have been instrumental in the completion of both.

And to my beloved John for his support and encouragement.

Preface

'... *when you can measure what you are speaking about, and express it in numbers, you know something about it; but when you cannot measure it, when you cannot express it in numbers, your knowledge is of a meagre and unsatisfactory kind; it may be the beginning of knowledge, but you have scarcely in your thoughts advanced to the state of* Science, *whatever the matter may be.'*

(Lord Kelvin, PLA, Vol. 1, Electrical Units of Measurement, 1883-05-03)

I find it hard to believe there was a time when measurement of observed performance of activity or of the impact of a disorder on patients/clients was not routinely quantified but I recall the early 1990s when this was the case; indeed for a small number of practitioners this is still the case. However, for the majority, standardized outcome measures have become an integral part of day-to-day practice.

For many individual practitioners, it is the prevailing measurement instruments in the service where he/she works which remain an integral part of practice and exposure to new versions and new instruments or outcome measures may be limited. This book takes five domains within rehabilitation and reviews a number of outcome measurement offerings. It does not make recommendations but reports what has been published to date so that the reader can make up his/her own mind.

Placing the systematic use of outcome measurement in clinical decision-making into a professional context illustrates how far we have come; nonetheless barriers to the use of outcome measures seem to be similar in all countries where such evaluation has been reported.

This book is mindful that readers may wish to explore for *new* instruments and outcome measures, which is why the chapters in Section 1 and 2 are included. Linking Chapter 2 in Section 1 with the tables in the relevant chapters in Section 3 and a review of the measures in Section 4 will, I hope, aid in the selection of new outcome measures in rehabilitation.

Instructions are included, where described, for each measurement instrument, nevertheless, in my experience, developers of instruments are very willing to answer questions about their application and the primary reference for each instrument will provide contact details. Web links are also provided so that readers can stay up-to-date with the developments in outcome measures as newer versions emerge.

Emma K. Stokes
2010

Section 1

Outcome measurement in context

This section introduces to you the developments in the use of outcome measurement in physiotherapy practice. This section is included to provide you with a context for where practice has come from, demonstrating the organic and responsive nature of practice internationally. It shows the similarity of experiences within different healthcare settings. It describes the International Classification of Functioning, Disability and Health (ICF) and how this can provide an internationally recognized taxonomy for describing health and health-related states. Links are provided to the World Confederation for Physical Therapy and its activities, which aim to inform the global physiotherapy community about ICF developments. Finally, this section provides some practical information about how you might go about choosing a new, or reviewing an existing, outcome measurement in your practice.

Outcome measurement and practice

1

CHAPTER CONTENTS

Introduction

In the past two decades, the focus of many healthcare policies and initiatives has been associated with the increased desire for both accountability and quality in healthcare (Kane 1997). The delivery of quality healthcare requires information on both the appropriateness of the intervention or management and its effectiveness. Kane (1994) suggests that appropriateness is informed by 'clear evidence of efficacy ... under a specified situation' and effectiveness requires the measurement of outcome – the two terms, he believes are not synonymous. Liebenson & Yeomans (1997) suggest that quality is demonstrated by improved outcomes and the utilization of evidence-based intervention. Bury & Mead (1998) employ the premise that clinical effectiveness encompasses evidence-based practice (EBP), and suggest that clinical effectiveness requires the

consideration of evidence in the context of external environmental and organizational influences. These represent just a fraction of the definitions used to illustrate a variety of terms employed in the language of healthcare evaluation. By defining each of these terms individually, the relationship between them may be fractured and it does not reflect the place of each and all in day-to-day clinical practice. Figure 1.1 illustrates the dynamic relationship that may exist between clinical effectiveness, evidence-based practice, clinical guidelines, outcomes research and the systematic use of standardized outcome measurement (sSOM).

Chapter outline

This chapter briefly considers the outcomes movement, evidence-based practice and clinical effectiveness in physiotherapy as a means of providing a context for the main review of outcome measurement in physiotherapy practice. This review considers the practice of standardized outcome measurement (SOM), the barriers reported to the systematic use of standardized outcome measures and the role of professional organizations in promoting and supporting sSOM.

The outcomes movement

In the late 1980s, Relman described the outcomes movement as the 'third revolution in medical care' (Relman 1988). In his opinion, the *Era of Expansion* came after the Second World War and continued

An individual patient/client presents to a physiotherapist (PT). The PT completes a full baseline assessment and set of appropriate outcome measurements. The PT then reviews the findings and outlines a proposed course of action, using the current version of clinical guidelines which is primarily based on professional consensus and which is appropriate to the clinical findings, and the preferences of the patient. At the following appointments, the PT re-evaluates the patient using standardized outcome measurement instruments, which demonstrate that the patient is improving. This is consistent with the reports of the patient. At the end of this period of intervention, the data (clinical, psychosocial, demographic characteristics, treatment, measured outcomes) gathered by the PT are entered into a database where, with the patients consent, it is used as part of a large formal outcomes study. This information along with that generated by other forms of research such as randomised controlled trials may form the basis of the evidence used to inform the development of clinical guidelines.

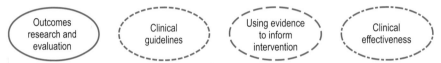

Figure 1.1 • The dynamic relationship that may exist between clinical effectiveness, evidence-based practice, clinical guidelines, outcomes research and the systematic use of standardized outcome measurement (sSOM).

until the late 1960s. This was followed by the *Era of Cost Containment*. He suggested that the third stage was the *Era of Assessment and Accountability*. The origins of this era are not completely clear (Kane 1997) but it is likely that a number of factors contributed. Large variations in the delivery of service, coupled with increasing expenditure, prompted questions about whether differences in outcome existed. With increasing amounts of national budgets being spent on healthcare, decisions about healthcare expenditure required information about the relative effectiveness of interventions and services, with a view to minimizing unnecessary expenditure – cost containment within the context of preserving quality of care. Managed care, with industrial accountability and productivity models, generated a revised way of thinking. Globally, the healthcare system had become a competitive marketplace. Individuals, insurance companies, health maintenance organizations, national health services and individual governments are all purchasers of healthcare. Market decisions are informed by outcomes of care (Epstein 1990, Jette 1995, Enderby & Kew 1995, Kane 1997, Hammond 2000, Beattie 2001).

Epstein (1990) described the three-fold effect of the outcomes movement on assessing outcomes. The emergence of a value placed on outcomes information had a subsequent impact on the way information is collected and stored. In some healthcare systems, large computerized databases are used to inform billing and reimbursement; while the presence of desktop computers in many departments and services has led to local analysis of data. This large-scale collection of data can be used to inform outcomes research and thus expand the existing knowledge base, working in tandem with the results of randomized controlled trials. The range of outcomes measured is broader. If health, as defined by the World Health Organization (1948): 'Health is a state of complete physical, mental and social well-being and not merely the absence of disease and infirmity', has become more measurable because of the development of well-constructed and evaluated measurement instruments (McDowell 2006), the outcomes movement has influenced the way that these outcome measures are used to inform practice and decision-making (Epstein 1990, Kane 1997).

Evidence-based practice

Evidence-based practice became the buzzword of the 1990s (Bury & Mead 1998), albeit that the origin of the concept is at least 150 years old (Sackett et al 1991); its emergence fuelled by increasing research activity and the desire to bring findings into practice and supported by published formats that made the information more accessible and advances in information technology. In physiotherapy, a long tradition of research does not exist, and a critical mass is still only emerging in some areas of practice and not present at all in others (Twomey 1996, Parry 1997). A number of factors have been cited as potential contributors to explain why some areas of healthcare do not have supporting evidence derived from research (Appleby et al 1995, Bury & Mead 1998):

- Difficulties in designing studies
- Difficulty in removing an intervention, which through custom and practice is now accepted, to perform a clinical trial
- Existing research that is of poor quality
- Randomized controlled trials not always appropriate to specific areas of healthcare
- Inadequate attention paid to the cost-effectiveness of interventions
- Failure to disseminate research findings.

In addition, specific factors in physiotherapy relate to the development of the profession, its historical placement under the auspices and protection of the medical profession (Roberts 1994, Parry 1995) and its lack of professional autonomy. In the UK, the profession grew out of the establishment of the Incorporated Society of Trained Masseuses in 1894 (Barclay 1994), which was later to become the Chartered Society of Physiotherapy. The practice of its members could only occur under doctor's orders. It was only in 1977 in the UK that physiotherapists finally gained professional autonomy and became first-contact practitioners. This occurred in the 1980s in other countries (Turner 2001). Prior to this there was a requirement for a referral from a medical practitioner, who also prescribed the treatment. The development of educational programmes for physiotherapy occurred in a non-uniform manner internationally. The USA had the first graduate programme (Moore 1995) in the 1920s, South Africa, Canada and Australia in the 1940s, 1950s and 1970s, respectively (Turner 2001). Despite the changes in the professional role, the emergence of a body of

graduates with research skills and equipped for the responsibility of autonomous practice and the drive for EBP in healthcare services, the use of research findings to inform the choice of treatment techniques is limited in physiotherapy (Turner 2001, Pomeroy & Tallis 2000). The factors that physiotherapists/physical therapists (PTs) use to inform treatment choice have been cited as original professional education, attendance at continuing professional development (CPD) courses, previous experience with a client or peer suggestion (Turner et al 1996, 1999, Carr et al 1994, Nilsson & Nordholm 1992). There is no mandate that requires the profession of physiotherapy to demonstrate efficacy of an intervention prior to its inclusion in an undergraduate course of study, or indeed in the area of continuing professional development (Stratford 1999). Often, in practice decisions are made on the basis of 'personal observations, precedence and consensus' (Parry 1997).

Across all aspects of healthcare, EBP initiatives, driven by the desire for creating greater consistency in the provision of services, have resulted in demands for and the development of Clinical Guidelines. This has presented and continues to present a challenge to many areas in healthcare provision, where a large body of evidence does not exist to support interventions and where professional consensus is hard to reach (Kane 1997, Stratford 1999). This is especially the case in physiotherapy because our research tradition is short but also because many 'higher' forms of research suggest that some physiotherapy interventions are ineffective or selectively effective (Stratford 1999, Pomeroy & Tallis 2000). Nevertheless, clinical guidelines exist in areas such as the management of osteoporosis, stress incontinence and soft tissue injury (CSP 1998, 1999, 2001b).

The use of outcome measures in practice

Significant challenges facing the physiotherapy profession with the emergence of the outcomes movement were the absence of an agreed framework for measurement and the absence of an ethos of using standardized measurement instruments. With respect to the latter, this chapter reviews the use of systematic outcomes measurement in physiotherapy practice under the following headings:

- The extent to which SOMs are employed in physiotherapy and related rehabilitation practice and the profile of this practice

- The attitudes towards use and the barriers identified by PTs in hindering the use of SOMs
- The role of professional organizations policy in promoting the use of SOM.

The information for the review in this chapter was obtained from a number of sources including a review of the published literature (Medline, CIHAHL and AMED).

Two methods are reported in the literature for the investigation of the extent to which standardized outcome measures are used in physiotherapy practice and rehabilitation: (1) survey instruments using self-report and (2) retrospective chart retrieval or chart audit. The first such reported work in physiotherapy was undertaken in 1992; a task force commissioned by the Canadian Physiotherapy Association and Health Canada completed a national survey, using a stratified random sample that examined the use of client outcome measures by PTs. The definition of an outcome measure was a 'published measurement scale'. The sample included individual practitioners and PT managers and was a random sample ($n = 309$) from a list of licensed therapists, with a response rate of approximately 80% (Mayo et al 1993, Cole et al 1995). The findings suggested that the use of standardized outcome measures was limited – 50% reported using the measures, but only 20% were able to identify one 'published measurement scale'. At the same time (the study was published 3 years after its completion), Chesson et al (1996) conducted a similar survey of PTs and occupational therapists (OTs) in Scotland. The survey participants were PT and OT managers in hospital and community-based departments. There was a 79% PT response, with only 44% of PT departments reporting to be using at least one standardized outcome measure, many of whom had only introduced the practice in the 1990s. Low rates of usage were reported in some regions suggesting the influence of local policy and SOMs more commonly used in the speciality of rehabilitation of older people than other specialities. Both studies suggested that the use of SOMs was emerging in physiotherapy practice. A pan-European review of the use of outcome measures was completed in 1998 (Torenbeek et al 2001). Using a postal questionnaire, 581 rehabilitation facilities in Germany, Ireland, Italy, Austria and the Netherlands were surveyed about a number of aspects of outcome measurement. The overall response rate was only 17.5% but the results are consistent the findings of the previous two surveys; the

authors concluded that, in the area of rehabilitation post stroke and for low back pain, systematic use of SOM is not yet common practice. The results identified that many of the measures used were 'neither published nor validated'. In a review of 182 rehabilitation centres in the UK, Turner-Stokes (1997) also noted that 77% of the centres represented by the respondents used at least one SOM. Stokes & O'Neill (1999, 2009) completed two surveys of practice in Ireland of physiotherapists working with older people and noted an increase in the use of SOMs in this area of practice over a period of 5 years from 1998 to 2003.

Retrospective chart retrieval and chart audit were the methods employed by Turner et al (1996, 1999) and Kirkness & Korner-Bitensky (2002). In 1993 in the UK, Turner et al (1996) screened a sample of case notes and included the case notes if pain was on the problem list, being treated or was noted in the initial assessment. A total of 1010 case notes were selected for audit. On initial assessment, 90% of cases presented with pain as a problem, 64% were treated for pain but only 21% actually quantified pain in any way. Reassessment occurred in 73% of cases and in those cases, 94% of cases had pain as a noted problem on reassessment. A total of 63% noted treatment for pain but only 2.5% quantified the pain on reassessment. Similar findings were reported in a later study by Turner et al (1999), in 1994–1996, 1,254 patient records were reviewed from five hospitals to consider the measurement of muscle strength and range of motion in the management of low back pain and after knee replacement surgery. A total of 810 charts met the criteria, i.e. the relevant parameter listed as a problem, in treatment plan, or treated by PT. In 95% of cases treatment for increasing muscle strength (MS) and range of motion (ROM) was documented. Both were initially quantified in approximately 64% of cases, but reassessment only took place in 10% of cases for MS and 30% for ROM. In both of these papers, charts from paediatric wards, patients <14 years, day hospitals for older people and patients aged >85 years were excluded. Nevertheless, the authors still noted that patients aged >55 years were less likely to have pain assessed than younger patients. Pain was measured using a body chart, and the end of range pain. MS was measured using manual muscle testing, limb girth and dynamometry. ROM was measured using goniometry. The attrition in the use of SOM across the period of intervention was noted by Kirkness & Korner-Bitensky (2002) in their investigation of the prevalence of

SOM use by PTs in the management of low back pain. They reviewed 256 randomly selected charts from 40 physiotherapy practice settings in Canada. The prevalence of PTs consistently using standardized outcome measures was low (34%). All but one of the respondents (53 PTs and 265 charts) employed measures of impairment of structures such as pain and range of motion, while one PT used a measure of activity limitation (disability). The authors divided their respondents into 'consistent users' and 'inconsistent users'. Clients of the former received more treatment sessions and were treated over a longer period of time; payment for their services was more likely to come from a hospital source as opposed to a private source or third party source, i.e. insurance company, workers' compensation scheme. The numeric pain rating score was the most commonly noted standardized measure employed, 27% used it at initial assessment but this level of usage dropped over the duration of intervention, with only 4% using it again at discharge. This attrition in the use of SOMs was consistent across all the instruments employed, suggesting that the information obtained was not used to measure change as a result of intervention.

In 2001, the results of a further survey on practice in Canada (completed in 1998) were published (Kay et al 2001). This survey focused on a review of practice following a number of strategic interventions by the Canadian Physiotherapy Association. In addition to general and specific questions on the use of outcome measurement, respondents were asked questions about their sources of information about outcome measurements and their confidence in a variety of situations relating to outcome measurement. In the second survey, respondents were identified as being either staff PTs ($n = 69$) or professional practice leaders (PPLs) ($n = 20$). Direct comparison could be made between the 1992 and 1998 surveys. A total of 41% ($n = 58$) of staff PTs reported that published measurement scales were used in their department in 1992, this increased by only 2% to 43%, ($n = 26$) in 1998. A more focused question asked respondents to consider a list of published outcome measures; check if they were familiar with the measure, and if they currently used it. Almost the entire sample reported that they currently used at least one of the outcome measures. The discrepancy between the two answers leading the authors to observe that 'it is difficult to conclude whether or not overall use of client outcome measures has increased since the 1990s'. It is interesting to note that two of the three stroke specific outcome measures reported as being used in 1992, were no longer reported as in use in the 1998 survey, although approximately one in three staff PTs and PPLs reported using the Chedoke McMaster Stroke Assessment Impairment Inventory Scale; an increase of 25%. The Berg Balance Scale was used by 45% of respondents ($n = 40$), an increase of 28% from 1992.

The five most frequently cited measures and the pattern of their use are outlined in Table 1.1. This question was not asked in the 1992 survey; hence no comparison of practice is available. The degree of attrition of use by OMs such as ROM, MS and pain is significantly less than that reported by Turner et al (1996, 1999) and Kirkness & Korner-Bitensky (2002), nevertheless one-third of PTs would still not measure balance, e.g. at both admission and discharge. These results indicate that optimum use of outcome measurements may not be occurring in clinical practice. This is consistent with the results of the section of the survey on the level of confidence in knowledge

Table 1.1 Standardized outcome measures used by Canadian physical therapists (% total)

Outcome measurement	Current use	At admission	At admission and discharge	More often
Range of motion	90	90	85	61
Manual muscle testing	88	92	85	68
Goal setting	73	95	85	57
Visual analogue scale pain	57	86	67	61
Berg Balance Scale	45	83	63	38

From Kay et al (2001).

Table 1.2 Confidence in the use of standardized outcome measures

Item	Staff PT		PPL	
	Mean ± SD	Range	Mean ± SD	Range
Knowing enough about test construction to develop own measure	27.8 ± 22.2	0–80	29.5 ± 21.4	0–80
Knowing how to link information to other information	45 ± 24.3	0–90	52 ± 22.4	10–90
Knowing how to compare scores to baseline levels across client groups	51.1 ± 25	0–100	54.8 ± 22.3	10–90
Knowing enough about measurement properties to choose	58.7 ± 21	10–90	64.5 ± 20.4	20–90
Knowing whether suitable measures are available	62.5 ± 22.7	10–100	73 ± 21.7	40–100
Knowing what to do with scores	62.9 ± 19.7	10–100	70 ± 22.9	10–90
Overall, knowing what to do with the information obtained	64 ± 21.6	10–100	68.5 ± 23.9	10–90
Knowing why to measure	71.5 ± 20	10–100	77.5 ± 23.4	10–100
Knowing how to track clients' progress with outcome measures	73 ± 16.2	20–100	73 ± 22	10–100
Knowing how to score measures	73.7 ± 16.2	20–100	75.5 ± 18.8	30–90
Knowing what to measure for client groups	73.8 ± 15.6	20–100	77.5 ± 23.1	0–100
Knowing how to administer OM in standardized manner	74.1 ± 16.3	20–100	75 ± 18.2	30–100
Total Confidence Score (higher score, greater confidence)	65.2 ± 14.2	10–100	68.5 ± 25.9	10–90

From Kay et al (2001).

about and use of SOMs. Respondents were asked to consider 12 statements and rate their confidence from 0% (not confident) to 100% (completely confident). Table 1.2 is a summary of the results reported. No statistically significant difference was noted between the groups for levels of confidence scores. The least amount of confidence was reported in the areas of measurement properties, linking information, comparing scores across groups and overall, what to do with the results. It would appear that outcome measures are used with confidence, but PTs are less confident or familiar with their broader use in the context of overall evaluation.

Attitudes and barriers to the use of SOM

Similar barriers to using outcome measures were reported in both Canadian surveys and were:

- *Lack of time*: reported by 52% staff PTs and 55% PPLs in 1998

- *Lack of knowledge about measures:* reported by 82% staff PTs and 75% PPLs in 1998
- *Limited availability of measures*: reported by 51% staff PTs and 50% PPLs in 1998
- *Not meeting needs of clients*: reported by 33% staff PTs and 60% PPLs in 1998
- *Lack of professional consensus on what to use*: reported by 27% staff PTs and 15% PPLs in 1998.

In addition to the quantitative survey results, the researchers undertook a series of focus groups to further examine the themes that had emerged following analysis of the survey (Huijbregts et al 2002). The results of this qualitative research methodology were supported by the quantitative survey results. It was observed that while it was accepted that the use of client outcome measures had become intrinsic in physiotherapy practice, consistent application was not uniform; and the utilization of the information gathered in a meaningful way lagged behind the collection of data. In terms of how practice is influenced, the authors noted that it is a combination of an organizational mandate to use standardized measures and the availability of an expert to advise on the outcomes evaluation that was required. To enhance practice in this area, the participants advocated that both employers and the professional organization needed to be proactively supportive. Enhanced communication with the developers of measurement instruments was repeatedly mentioned as a way of optimizing the subsequent use of newly developed outcome measures. Consistent with the survey results, limiting factors reported were insufficient knowledge, time constraints, lack of equipment, accessibility of forms and space, e.g. for timed walks. Kirkness & Korner-Bitensky (2002), although their methodology differed from that of the previous authors, also noted that barriers such as limited knowledge of instruments and their development; time; failure of the instruments to meet client needs; and lack of consensus on what to use were all reported by respondents. Russek et al (1997) investigated the attitudes of PTs and OTs to standardized data collection and the characteristics of the therapists that inform these attitudes. Standardized evaluation forms designed for an orthopaedic patient population were provided to all clinics that agreed to participate. These included three principle forms: (1) a data collection tool (DCT) for initial and subsequent re-evaluation, (2) daily treatment forms and (3) discharge status forms. Both videotapes and written instructions were provided for the measurements that formed part of the data collection tool. A number of measurements were included – for shoulder, elbow, knee, foot and ankle – but only those appropriate to each specific client needed to be used. Completed datasets were sent to a central site where the information could be entered on a computer. Information about attitudes and personal demographic data was gathered through a 67-item questionnaire. Principle-axis factor analysis (on 33 items) yielded five factors that accounted for 42.5% of the total variability, namely:

1. Inconvenience associated with the completion of the data collection tool, i.e. initial and re-evaluation
2. Acceptance of operational definitions – the instructions given for the various measurements that were performed as part of the evaluation
3. Automation – the usefulness of computers with respect to gathering and processing this type of information
4. Daily treatment forms – issues specifically surrounding the use and impact of the daily treatment forms
5. Training.

Two-thirds of respondents to the questionnaire reported that they had 'studied thoroughly' the operational definitions for at least one body part included in the study. Nonetheless, reported participation rate for completing and submitting one complete dataset was only 50%. The extent to which the latter activity occurred was significantly associated with those respondents who identified research as a professional goal. This was also significantly associated with factor 2 (acceptance of operational definitions). Increased numbers of datasets completed and submitted were both significantly associated with factors 2 and 5 – comfort with operational definitions and adequate training. The inconvenience associated with the DCTs was significantly associated with greater client numbers per day. The authors conclude that adequate training in operational definitions of measures and data collection will enhance participation in systematic use of measures but that this needs to occur in the context of optimizing the method of data gathering, perhaps through the provision of automated patient reports. In the European survey, it was interesting to note that the degree to which collected data was processed statistically later varied from country to country, with Ireland the lowest at 17% and Germany the highest at 90%. This may reflect the reason why the outcomes data is gathered; statistical processing of the data occurs most often in countries where the information is gathered for the purposes of quality management and informing providers and policy-makers. Greater skill and knowledge of how gathered SOM data may be used at a later stage to inform practice would perhaps influence more consistent measurement practice.

The role of professional organizations in promoting the systematic use of SOMs

The Chartered Society of Physiotherapy (CSP), which is the representative body for physiotherapists within the UK and the Canadian Physiotherapy Association (CPA) have both completed significant work in this area of development. In 2004, the Council of the CSP adopted a strategy (CSP 2004) with its focus on research and clinical effectiveness which built on its first such strategy published in 1999. As part of the achievements of the work incorporated in these strategies, the one that focused specifically on SOM was the development of an outcome measures database (Hammond 1999). This provides information about the measurement properties of a large range of outcome measurements. A number of clinical guidelines have been developed and within those documents are suggestions for which standardized measurements should be used in practice, e.g. osteoporosis and incontinence (CSP 1999, 2001b). Two documents are designed specifically to provide information on SOMs, one deals with depression (CSP 2002) and the other, low back pain related functional limitation (CSP 2001a). Additional national networking activities have been created with Clinical Interest Groups and these activities have been ongoing (Hammond 2000). To date, no formal evaluation of the impact of these measures has been completed.

The Canadian Physiotherapy Association (CPA) has clearly described the process and progress their organization has made to enhance the systematic use of outcome measurements. Their definition of evidence-based practice as 'practice which has a theoretical body of knowledge, uses the best available scientific evidence in clinical decision making and uses standardized outcome measures to evaluate the care provided' is unique, in that it includes an emphasis on the use of standardized outcome measures (Parker-Taillon 2002). The CPA EBP initiatives include activities in six key areas:

1. Entry-level Curriculum Guidelines will be developed which promote the development of evidence-based practitioners
2. Access to high quality, recognized continuing professional development that promotes and supports EBP will be available to Canadian PTs
3. Clinical practice guidelines and strategies for their implementation, which will promote EBP and assist in clinical decision-making will be developed
4. CPA Accreditation Programme will be revised to promote EBP and support such practice
5. Outcome Measures. Canadian PTs are expected to consistently use standardized outcome measures in their daily practice
6. A database will be developed which will examine the effectiveness and efficiency of Canadian PT services.

The European Region of the World Confederation for Physical Therapy adopted a series of Core Standards in May 2002 (ER-WCPT, 2002). Standard 6 reads as follows: 'Taking account of the patient's problems, a published, standardized, valid, reliable and responsive outcome measure is used to evaluate the change in the patient's health status.' The standard is

---

Box 1.1

European Region of the World Confederation for Physical Therapy

Core Standards

Standard 6: taking account of the patient's problems, a published, standardized, valid, reliable and responsive outcome measure is used to evaluate the change in the patient's health status

- Criteria 6.1: The physiotherapist selects an outcome measure that is relevant to the patient's problem
- Criteria 6.2: The physiotherapist ensures the outcome measure is acceptable to the patient. The physiotherapist selects an outcome measure that he/ she has the necessary skill and experience to use, administer and interpret
- Criteria 6.6: The result of the measurement is recorded immediately
- Criteria 6.7: The same measure is used at the end episode of care.

---

listed in Box 1.1. The ER-WCPT adopted the Core Standards in 2002 and the expectation is that each of the member organizations will adopt the Standards for their own country.

Summary

It is accepted that the systematic use of standardized outcome measures is required in physiotherapy practice. This requires a commitment from individual practitioners, the organizations where they work and the professional physiotherapy organizations. The extent to which SOMs are used may be influenced by an organizational mandate, but there still appears to be a lack of understanding as to why SOMs are useful; this is reflected in the attrition that occurs after the initial measure is taken at baseline. To fully understand the relevance of outcomes data, the individual has to be equipped with the relevant knowledge and ability to interpret measurement properties (see Chs. 4, 5 & 6). It appears from the literature review that the 1990s have been a period of significant change in practice, with increasing numbers of PTs using SOMs. The future of this practice in the coming years will be to optimize this practice with a view to enhancing individual clinical decision-making and broader outcomes research.

References

Appleby J, Walshe K, Ham C: *Acting on the evidence A review of clinical effectiveness; sources of information, dissemination and implementation,* Birmingham, 1995, National Association of Health Authorities and Trusts.

Barclay J: *In good hands. The history of the Chartered Society of Physiotherapy 1894–1994,* Oxford, 1994, Butterworth Heinemann.

Beattie P: Measurement of health outcomes in the clinical setting: applications to physiotherapy, *Physiother Theory Pract* 17:173–185, 2001.

Bury T, Mead J: *Evidence-based healthcare: A practical guide for therapists,* Oxford, 1998, Butterworth Heinemann.

Carr JH, Mungovan SF, Shepherd RB, et al: Physiotherapy in stroke rehabilitation: basis for Australian physiotherapists choice of treatment, *Physiother Theory Pract* 10:201–209, 1994.

Chartered Society of Physiotherapy: *Clinical guidelines for the management of soft tissue injury with PRICE,* 1998. Online. Available: www.csp.org.uk/effectivepractice/ clinicalguidelines/ physiotherapyguidelines.cfm#4.

Chartered Society of Physiotherapy: *Clinical guidelines for the management of osteoporosis,* 1999. Online. Available: www.csp.org.uk/ effectivepractice/clinicalguidelines/ physiotherapyguidelines.cfm#4.

Chartered Society of Physiotherapy: *Low back pain-related functional measures. CLEF4,* 2001a. Online. Available: www.csp.org.uk/ effectivepractice/outcomemeasures/ publications.cfm?id.

Chartered Society of Physiotherapy: *Clinical guidelines for the management of stress urinary incontinence,* 2001b. Online. Available: www.csp.org.uk/ effectivepractice/clinicalguidelines/ physiotherapyguidelines.cfm#4.

Chartered Society of Physiotherapy: *Outcome measures for people with depression (a working document) CLEF5,* 2002. Online. Available: www.csp.org.uk/effectivepractice/ outcomemeasures/publications.cfm? id.

Chartered Society of Physiotherapy: *Research and clinical effectiveness strategy,* London, 2004, CSP. Online. Available: www.csp.org.uk/director/ members/libraryandpublications/ csppublications.cfm? item_id=74C872AAB5940758 2BCB78248F1B67AC 17.06.2008.

Chesson R, MacLeod M, Massie S: Outcome measures used in therapy departments in Scotland, *Physiotherapy* 82(12):673–679, 1996.

Cole B, Finch E, Gowland C, et al: Basmajian J, editor: *Physical rehabilitation outcome measures,* Baltimore, 1995, Williams and Wilkins.

Enderby P, Kew E: Outcome measurement in physiotherapy using the WHO's Classification of Impairment, *Disability and Handicap* 81(4):177–180, 1995.

Epstein A: The outcomes movement – will it get us where we want to go? *N Engl J Med* 323:266–270, 1990.

European Region of the World Confederation for Physical Therapy: *European Core Standards of Physiotherapy Practice,* 2002. Online. Available: www.physio-europe.org/ index.php?action=19 Accessed June 19, 2009.

Hammond R: Why an outcome measures database? *Physiotherapy* 85(5): 234–235, 1999.

Hammond R: Evaluation of physiotherapy by measuring the outcome, *Physiotherapy* 86(4): 170–172, 2000.

Huijbregts MPJ, Myers AM, Kay TM, et al: Systematic outcome measurement in clinical practice: challenges experiences by physiotherapists, *Physiother Can* 54:25–31, 36, 2002.

Jette AM: Outcomes research: shifting the dominant research paradigm in physical therapy, *Phys Ther* 75 (11):965–970, 1995.

Kane R: Looking for physical therapy outcomes, *Phys Ther* 74:425–429, 1994.

Kane R: *Understanding healthcare outcomes,* Maryland, 1997, Aspen.

Kay TM, Myers AM, Huijbregts MPJ: How far have we come since 1992? A comparative survey of physiotherapists' use of outcome measures, *Physiother Can* 53:268–275, 281, 2001.

Kirkness C, Korner-Bitensky N: Prevalence of outcome measure use by physiotherapists in the management of low back pain, *Physiother Can* 54(4):249–257, 2002.

Liebenson C, Yeomans S: Outcomes assessment in musculoskeletal medicine, *Man Ther* 2(2):67–74, 1997.

Mayo N, Cole B, Dowler J, et al: Use of outcome measurement in physiotherapy: Survey of current practice, *Can J Rehabil* 7:81–83, 1993.

McDowell I: *Measuring Health. A Guide to Rating Scales and Questionnaires,* ed 3, New York, 2006, Oxford University Press.

Moore W: *Healing the generations: a history of physical therapy and the American Physical Therapy Association,* Connecticut, 1995, Greenwich Publishing.

Nilsson LM, Nordholm LA: Physical therapy in stroke rehabilitation: Basis for Swedish therapists choice of treatment, *Physiother Theory Pract* 8:49–55, 1992.

Parker-Taillon D: CPA initiatives put the spotlight on evidence-based practice in physiotherapy, *Physiother Can* Winter 24:12–15, 2002.

Parry A: Ginger Rogers did everything that Fred Astaire did backwards and in high heels, *Physiotherapy* 81(6): 310–319, 1995.

Parry A: New paradigms for old: musings on the shape of clouds, *Physiotherapy* 83(8):423–433, 1997.

Pomeroy V, Tallis R: Physical therapy to improve movement performance and functional ability post stroke. Part 1: Existing evidence, *Rev Clin Gerontol* 10:261–290, 2000.

Relman AS: Assessment and accountability: the third revolution in medical care, *N Engl J Med* 319:1220–1222, 1988.

Roberts P: Theoretical models of physiotherapy, *Physiotherapy* 80 (6):361–366, 1994.

Russek L, Wooden M, Ekedahl S, Bush A: Attitudes toward standardised data collection, *Phys Ther* 77(7):714–728, 1997.

Sackett DL, Haynes RB, Guyatt GH, et al: *Clinical epidemiology. A basic science for clinical medicine*, ed 3, Boston, 1991, Little, Brown.

Stokes EK, O'Neill D: The use of standardised assessments by physiotherapists, *Brit J Ther Rehabil* 6(11):560–565, 1999.

Stokes EK, O'Neill D: Use of outcome measures in physiotherapy practice in Ireland from 1998 to 2003 and comparison to Canadian trends, *Physiother Can* 60:109–116, 2009.

Stratford P: Who will decide the efficacy of physiotherapeutic interventions? *Physiother Can* Fall:235–236, 238, 1999.

Torenbeek M, Caulfield B, Garrett M, et al: Current use of outcome measures for stroke and low back pain rehabilitation in five European countries: first results of the ACROSS project, *Int J Rehabil Res* 24:95–101, 2001.

Turner PA, Whitfield A, Brewster S, et al: The assessment of pain: an audit of physiotherapy practice, *Aust J Physiother* 42(1):55–62, 1996.

Turner PA, Harby-Owen H, Shackleford F, et al: Audits of physiotherapy practice, *Physiother Theory Pract* 15:261–274, 1999.

Turner P: Evidence-based practice and physiotherapy in the 1990s, *Physiother Theory Pract* 17:107–121, 2001.

Turner-Stokes L, Turner-Stokes T: The use of standardised outcome measures in rehabilitation centres in the UK, *Clin Rehabil* 11:306–313, 1997.

Twomey L: Editorial – research, more essential than ever, *Physiother Res Int* 1(2):iii–iiv, 1996.

World Health Organization: Constitution. In WHO, editor: *Basic documents*, Geneva, 1948, WHO.

International classification of functioning, disability and health (ICF)

2

CHAPTER CONTENTS

Introduction

The constitution of the World Health Organization mandates the production of international classifications on health with a view to having a framework that is based on consensus and is both useful and meaningful to assist governments, providers and consumers in providing a common language.

The classifications are described as reference classifications and derived classifications, the former including the International Classification of Diseases (ICD) and the International Classification of Functioning, Disability and Health (ICF), and the latter including the International Classification of Diseases for Oncology, 3rd edn. (ICD-O-3). The purpose of the WHO Family of International Classifications (WHO-FIC) is to promote the appropriate selection of classifications in the range of settings in the health field across the world.

In May 2001, the World Health Assembly endorsed the International Classification of Functioning, Disability and Health.

Chapter outline

The purpose of this chapter is to acquaint the reader with the International Classification of Functioning, Disability and Health (ICF) (WHO 2001) and to understand how it can be used in the context of measurement. Links will be provided to established Core Sets of the ICF for various conditions. In addition, linking rules for existing outcome measures will be discussed.

What is ICF?

ICF is a classification system, the overall aim of which is to 'provide unified and standard language and framework for the description of health and health related states' (WHO 2001). As a classification instrument, it can be used in rehabilitation and outcome evaluation. It considers health and health related states in two parts: (1) Functioning and Disability and (2) Contextual Factors.

Part 1 has the following components:

- Body functions: physiological functions of the body systems
- Body structures: anatomical parts of the body such as organs, limbs and their components
- Activity: execution of a task or action by an individual
- Participation: involvement in a life situation.

Impairments are problems in body function or structure considered to be a significant deviation or loss. Activity limitations are difficulties an individual may have in carrying out activities and restrictions in participation are problems an individual may experience

DOI: 10.1016/B978-0-443-06915-4.00002-4

Table 2.1 The International Classification of Functioning, Disability and Health (ICF) (WHO 2001)

Definitions of components of ICF	ICF domains	ICF categories	Definition of categories
Impairments are problems with body functions and/or structures.	Body functions – physiological functions	b110 Consciousness functions	State of awareness and alertness
	Body functions – sensory functions and pain	b280 Pain	Sensation of pain
	Body functions – movement functions	b7651 Tremor	Functions of alternating contraction and relaxation of a group of muscles around a joint
	Body structures – structures of the brain	s1103	Basal ganglia and related structures
Limitations in activity are difficulties associated with performing an activity. Restrictions in participation are challenges that a person may have in a life situation.	Activities and participation – mobility	d410 Changing basic body position	Getting into and out of a body position and moving from one location to another
	Activities and participation – carrying, moving and handling objects	d430 Lifting and carrying objects	Raising up an object or taking something from one place to another
	Activities and participation	d450 Walking	Moving along a surface on foot

in involvement in life situations. Table 2.1 provides some examples of ICF domains and categories and codes within the domains. Within functions, structures and activities and participation, there are extensive lists of categories, some of which may be applicable to the groups of patients seen in your practice and others which may not be applicable.

Part 2, the contextual factors, includes environmental factors external to individuals that may have either a positive or negative impact on the individual. Personal factors are not classified by the ICF.

ICF Core Sets are sets of categories that apply to particular patient groups or conditions and have been developed using rigorous professional consensus techniques involving international experts. The ICF Research Branch (2008) website provides information about the ongoing research work in this area. Examples of Core Sets that have been developed are for stroke, breast cancer, rheumatoid arthritis, osteoporosis, osteoarthritis, diabetes, low back pain and obesity. Those under development include spinal cord injury, manual medicine, and multiple sclerosis. Core sets may be considered the 'minimal standards for the reporting of functioning and health (Cieza et al 2005). If there is a Core Set for your area of practice, its contents can be used to describe the

status of your client/patient group. The value of ICF is that it is an international language that allows pan-European and international comparisons of health and the state of health.

What does the ICF aim to do?

The ICF aims to:

* Provide a scientific basis for understanding and studying health and health related states as well as the outcomes of interventions and the determinants of health
* Establish a common language for describing health and health related states with a view to improving communication
* Allow for the comparison of data across countries, disciplines, services and time
* Provide systematic coding for health information systems.

How can I use the ICF in practice?

The ICF provides a system of quantification for each component, e.g. in the case of d410, changing basic body position, see Table 2.2.

Table 2.2 The ICF system of quantification (e.g. case d410)

ICF coding	Descriptive interpretation	% loss
d410.0 – No problem	(none, absent, neglible, . . .)	0–4
d410.0 – Mild problem	(slight, low, . . .)	5–24
d410.0 – Moderate problem	(medium, fair, . . .)	25–49
d410.0 – Severe problem	(high, extreme, . . .)	50–95
d410.0 – Complete problem	(total, . . .)	96–100
d410.8 – Not specified		
d410.0 – Not applicable		

The WHO (2001) states that 'for this quantification to be used in a universal manner, assessment procedures need to be developed through research. Broad ranges of percentages are provided for those cases in which calibrated assessment instruments or other standards are available to quantify the impairment, capacity limitations, performance problem or barrier.'

The mechanism for estimating the extent of a limitation may be self-reported or another measurement system can be used to estimate the level of limitation as described above. Linking ICF categories with standardized outcome measurements is not precise and linking rules have been developed. Eight linking rules have been described (Cieza et al 2005) (Table 2.3).

Table 2.3 Outline of the eight linking rules

Linking rules	Example of application to Berg Balance Scale
Before links are made between the concepts contained within an existing outcome measure and the ICF, those involved in linking should be very familiar with the ICF.	
Each meaningful concept within the OM is linked to the most precise ICF category.	In the Berg Balance Scale (BBS), there are 12 items. It is possible to link 10 to ICF Sitting to standing – d4103 Sitting Standing unsupported – d4154 Maintaining a standing position Sitting with back unsupported – d4153 Maintaining a sitting position Standing to sitting – d4104 Standing Transfers – d4200 Transferring oneself while sitting Reaching forward – d4106 Shifting the body's centre of gravity Pick up object – d4105 Bending
Do not use the description categories 'other specified'. Do not use the description categories 'other unspecified'.	For example, with the BBS the items about turning 360 degrees and placing one foot on a stool could be 'd429 Changing and maintaining body position, other specified and unspecified' but this is not correct
If an item within the OM does not provide sufficient detail for it to be linked with an ICF category it is assigned 'not definable' (nd).	
If an item within the OM is not contained within the ICF categories it is assigned 'not covered' (nc).	
If an item within the OM is a personal factor as defined by the ICF, it is assigned 'personal factor' (pf).	
If an item within the OM relates to a health condition or diagnosis, it is assigned 'health condition' (hc).	

Why is the ICF important in my practice?

The ICF can be used to measure clinical outcomes as described above. But it can also be used to describe the health or health related state of users of your service; this description may be useful for you when describing your service, when comparing your service with another one that uses the same ICF descriptors and when assessing if your service actually matches the needs of the services users. It is a language that is accessible and understandable to all members of the multidisciplinary team, to the commissioners of services and indeed to the users of services.

International teams are working on Core Sets and you, as a specialist can be involved in the development of such Core Sets. The invitation may come through your professional organization via the World Confederation for Physical Therapy.

World Confederation for Physical Therapy and ICF

The World Confederation for Physical Therapy is the sole international voice for physical therapy. It represents more than 300 000 physical therapists worldwide through its 101 member organizations. WCPT is committed to forwarding the physical therapy profession and its contribution to global health. It encourages high standards of physical therapy research, education and practice. As part of its mission and strategic plans, WCPT aims to raise the profile of the ICF with the members of WCPT; it also works with WHO on collaborative work to encourage and gain greater use of the ICF by physiotherapists. WCPT has a network for ICF, which enables physiotherapists to share the experiences of using ICF. It also has links to other helpful ICF information (WCPT 2009).

References

Cieza A, Geyh S, Chatterji S, et al: ICF linking rules: an update based on lessons learned, *J Rehabil Med* 37:212–218, 2005.

ICF Research Branch: *Research: Branch & Co-operation projects*, 2008. Online

Available: www.icf-research-branch. org. Accessed June 16, 2009.

WCPT: *Global Health – ICF. World Confederation for Physical Therapy*, 2009. Online. Available: www.wcpt. org/icf. Accessed June 16, 2009.

WHO: *International Classification of Functioning, Disability and Health*, Geneva, 2001, World Health Organization.

How to choose an outcome measure

3

Introduction

At some point in your career you may be asked to choose an outcome measure. It may be because you have reviewed your current arrangements and believe that the current practice should be updated or it may be because you are starting a new service. The temptation when starting out in clinical outcome measurement is to jump straight to the measures and to try to work out which ones to use. Throughout this book, a more focused approach is suggested as this will help you to avoid common traps and pitfalls, to help you avoid wasting time and energy, and to try to make the process of outcome measurement productive, meaningful and of value.

Chapter outline

The purpose of this chapter is to assist in the choice of an outcome measurement and its subsequent use in practice. It is a step-by-step guide to choosing and using outcome measurements in day-to-day clinical practice. It includes a short consideration of setting-up the project management of seeking a new or different outcome measure and a model for evaluating outcome measures that may seem appropriate for use in your practice or service as, when you search for outcome measures, a number may be available which measure the same or similar concepts.

A roadmap

Box 3.1 illustrates a roadmap of the process which may be of assistance when starting out. You may already be using outcome measures (OMs) and need assistance with knowing what to do with the results. Or you may be starting out to see which OM will be most suitable for your practice.

© 2011, Elsevier Ltd.
DOI: 10.1016/B978-0-443-06915-4.00003-6

Project manage the process of choosing and using OMs

If you are starting off the process of choosing outcome measures for your patients, clients, service or practice, you might like to think of the choice and subsequent use as a stand-alone project initially. It is always helpful to define the team who will be involved in the choice of OM, it could be just one person but often it will involve a number of colleagues. Describe your plan with aims and objectives and clearly identify the expected outcome. Other aspects of the project will be identifying the resources, if any, that are required. For example:

- Staffing
  - What are the skills and abilities required to complete different tasks?
  - Who has these?
  - Are they able to complete within the timescales?
- Costs
  - Staffing
  - Meetings
  - Other, e.g. purchase of measure, training, stationery.

You may also wish to consider the potential things that could arise which might hinder or disrupt successful completion of the project. Identifying these risks is useful because it may help to prevent them becoming problematic, or at least, alert you to the need to look for help. Questions you might wish to consider are:

- What are the risks involved in delivering this project?
- How can they be managed?
- What contingency plans are needed?

Communication will be important both for the project team and the end-users of the OM. You may wish to consider the questions listed below before you commence.

- What will be done to ensure members of the team know what is expected of them and when, what others outside the team are expected to do and when, and what quality is necessary?
- Who is the target audience?
- Who has a stake in this project?
- What needs to be in place in order to retain their commitment to the project?
- Who will keep them informed of progress?

Someone should be charged with being the day-to-day project manager; taking responsibility for moving the project along, ensuring people deliver what they say they will, and to agreed timescales and quality, etc. This can be supported by having project stages and agreed critical points to aid monitoring and assessment of progress. It might also be helpful to have in place an agreed process to decide whether the project is on track or not, and if not why and what needs to be done to resolve this. Finally, evaluation of the project should also include recommendations and a plan for review.

Box 3.2 and Table 3.1 illustrate an example of how this might work.

It is also helpful to identify who will take responsibility for each objective and what the overall time line of the project will be (Table 3.1).

This is proposed because it can overcome problems with data collation (e.g. they hadn't identified beforehand what they would do with data collected); colleague engagement (because they hadn't agreed why and how they were going to collect data); and confusion (because they didn't make clear decisions at the start as to what the information was for).

Success in selecting a measure will mean:

Box 3.2

Project plan – patient satisfaction survey

Project team

Mary Jones (Clinical Specialist), Sam Chari (Senior PT), Nora Clare (Senior PT), Tom Shaw (Staff PT), Sarah Byrne (Administrator), Larry Murphy and Lara Santisteban (recent patients of the service, now discharged who agreed to review the OM).

Aim

To search for, evaluate and choose a patient satisfaction survey instrument for use with patients referred with low back pain to the physiotherapy service.

Objectives

1. To search the relevant literature and other sources for patient satisfaction surveys
2. To identify a number of possible surveys
3. To review the surveys and decide if they are suitable for our service
4. To make a decision on which to use
5. To prepare a presentation for the department on the use of the OM including information on how the measurements can inform individual decision-making and also how the data will contribute to the overall department
6. To create a simple mechanism for gathering the data, inputting it into spreadsheets and analysing it to create departmental reports
7. To establish a pilot period of use of the OM and evaluate the project thereafter and report back to all staff.

Table 3.1 Task allocation for project to select OM

What	Who	When
To search the relevant literature for patient satisfaction surveys – library search	Mary Jones (MJ) and Sam Chari (SC) Liaise with library staff and academic department	January 2009–March 2009
To search the relevant literature for patient satisfaction surveys – other sources	Nora Clare (NC), Tom Shaw (TS) and Lara Santisteban (LS) Liaise with patient organizations and other departments	January 2009–March 2009
To identify a number of possible surveys	MJ, SC, NC, TS	End March 2009
To review the surveys and decide if they are suitable for our service	All	April 2009
To make a decision on which to use	All	End April 2009
To prepare a presentation for the department	MJ, SB, LM	May 2009
To create a simple mechanism for gathering the data, inputting it into spreadsheets and analysing it to create departmental reports	SB	April 2009
To evaluate the project thereafter and report back to all staff	All	End December 2009

- Individual clinicians and users experiencing the evaluation of practice as a constructive and enabling process that they understand, enjoy and that contributes to their professional development
- The project is seen through to completion with the planned outputs that are fit for their intended purpose and are used by the target audience.

How do I choose a measure to use in my clinical practice?

The measures you choose will be informed by your answer to these questions: Why do I want to measure? What is the purpose of the evaluation?

Because it is best practice

The World Confederation for Physical Therapy in its Position Statement on Patient Documentation (WCPT 2009), the European Core Standards of Physiotherapy (ER-WCPT 2002) and indeed other national and international standards, require that a standardized outcome measure is used in your practice. So you may simply be collecting information to help you make decisions about individual clients or patients, or you may have to collect the information for an external stakeholder.

To help you as a clinician see the effect of your treatment

You have an internal drive to evaluate the effectiveness of practice on a personal level but on more careful consideration, the issues you are really thinking about could be:

- 'I want to see if I am getting the results I should'
- 'I want to see if I am being clinically effective'
- 'I want to monitor and review progress in an objective manner'
- 'I want to use a measure to help motivate my patient'.

To provide information for you to give to a third party

Another reason comes from an external source; you have been asked to do it! This might be from a fellow professional, e.g. physiotherapist, doctor, occupational therapist; a patient, insurance company, a commissioner of services or a manager.

The question they might ask is:

- 'I've heard physiotherapy is good for people with a bad back, show me how good this practice is at treating this condition'
- 'Why should we commission physiotherapy, what success do you get?'
- 'Why do we need to keep treating this patient?'

A physiotherapy manager is likely to be responding to a request to demonstrate value for money for the service they manage.

What is the purpose of evaluation?

There are a variety of reasons for wanting to measure. Arguably the prime one for physiotherapists is to evaluate how much their patients do or do not change. However, other reasons exist: to define the role of physiotherapeutic exercise with this population, to help patients see how they are changing, to provide information to team members and those securing the delivery of services of the impact of physiotherapeutic exercise. Feinstein (1987) suggests that the purpose of measurement is the description of a state, a measure of change, the estimation of prognosis and to offer a guideline. In addition, an OM can:

- Assist in the development of a problem list
- Denote a change due to intervention
- Predict an outcome
- Be used as a teaching tool
- Be a communication aid with other services.

Measuring change

Commonly in clinical practice, you must establish baseline information at the beginning of treatment in a reliable manner, and re-test the same domains at the end of intervention. You may also wish to predict an end-point, e.g. return to work or risk of falls. To do this in a valid way, you should identify, and agree with the patient, the aims of intervention. These aims may vary with each individual patient. The reason for evaluation and for whom the information is collected should be clearly identified before deciding on what measures to use. Physiotherapists should do this with an awareness of the work of other clinicians in the team, e.g. if a specific measure of depression is being collected by another team member, then the results of this can be used by the physiotherapist. Using a different measure in this circumstance would be inappropriate.

Consider this question: What am I attempting to change? In general, the answer might be to speed up recovery or maintain a functional status; it may be to provide support, education, advice, or practical problem-solving to a formal or informal carer; it might be to deliver a planned programme of activity or an intervention to a specific population. To help choose a measure, consider this question in more depth; what is it about recovery or functional status that you want to speed up or maintain? This could be a patient's ability to cope, their self-esteem, confidence, sleep patterns, an impairment, improved ability to do something, or to participate in day-to-day life, or another of the many aims of physiotherapy healthcare. Once you have identified your aims of treatment, it will be easier to decide how you will record whether you succeed or not.

Different types of measures

'Generic' health status measures 'assess overall health status, including social, emotional, and physical health status, and are intended to be applicable across a broad spectrum of diseases, interventions, and demographic and cultural subgroups' (Binkley et al 1999). One example is the SF-36. 'Disease-' and 'condition-specific' measures assess the patient's perception of a specific disease or health problem; these measures might be patient-completed, some are clinician-completed, and some are for the family or carers to complete. An example of a disease-specific measure for use with patients who have osteo-arthritis is the Arthritis Impact Measurement II scales (Meenan et al 1980). In addition, using the ICF categories as a framework (see Ch. 2), some measures focus on measuring body structures and functions and others consider activities and participation (see Table 2.1). Careful consideration should be given to only using measures of impairment such as range of motion or strength as for many patients and clients changes on these measures may not translate into any real functional change and for external audiences, such as other healthcare professionals or managers, they may not be meaningful. They can be very useful in planning components of treatment intervention but for meaningful change to be captured, outcome measures should focus on activities and participation.

Where do I find outcome measures?

Section 3 in this book will provide you with details of many outcome measures but the section is not exhaustive. It also tries not to replicate details that may be reported in other books. Obtaining a measure can be difficult. Identifying articles is tricky and once found, papers can be of varying quality and information on the properties of the measure either non-existent or conflicting. Many papers of relevance do not identify the specific outcome measure in the title, summary, or in keywords. Another problem is that copyright restrictions on instruments are variable. Some measures can be used freely, others can be used with the author's permission for free and other measures can only be obtained and used by paying a fee. However, if you have carefully considered the purpose

for evaluation, who the information is for, and what the aim of intervention is, choosing, appraising and rejecting a measure should be less complicated.

Assessing the quality of a measure

Initially, there are three basic questions to answer:

- Has it been published in a peer-reviewed journal?
- Is it standardized?
- Is there a written scoring procedure?

If the answer is 'no' to any of these questions, then the value of the measure is questionable.

Has it been published?

A measurement property may have papers published about its measurement properties but unfortunately this does not always mean it is publically available. Some OMs are published with the paper, e.g. the Lower Extremity Function Scale (Binkley et al 1999); others are available on websites, e.g. the Disabilities of Arm, Shoulder and Hand outcome measure (DASH) (IHW 2009) whereas others are available by contacting the authors, e.g. Multi-Dimensional Fatigue Inventory MFI-20 (Smets et al 1995). Some measures are protected by copyright, e.g. Functional Assessment of Multiple Sclerosis (FAMS) (Cella et al 1996). This means you need to get permission to use them. You may have to pay for this.

Is it standardized?

Standardization procedures should provide clear, explicit instructions on how to undertake every part of the measure. This may be presented in the original article, e.g. Knee Injury and Osteoarthritis Outcome Score (KOOS) (Roos et al 1998), or a manual may be required, e.g. Prosthetic Profile of the Amputee (PPA) (Grise et al 1993).

Does it have clear scoring instructions?

A measure may have a few scoring requirements, e.g. Functional Ambulation Categories (Holden et al 1994). With this measure, the administrator categorizes the patient into one of five defined scores. Other measures adopt a slightly more sophisticated scoring system, e.g. Adelaide Activities Profile (Clark and Bond 1995). Each answer is compared to a scoring card that gives a weighted number. The scores for each answer are then added together. For measures with more sophisticated procedures and scoring methods, training may be required. This could be in the form of internet online help, half day, full day, or longer courses, e.g. Treatment Evaluation by Le Roux Method (TELER) (Le Roux 1993).

If the answer to these three questions is 'yes', then you should now consider the measurement *properties* of the measure. This essentially involves consideration of how well the measure has been devised, how successfully it will help you answer the question 'can I trust the results I get from using the measure', and how feasible it is for you to use in your daily working life.

How do I know if a measure is any good?

An outcome measure should be standardized, with explicit instructions for administration and scoring. A measure should be reliable, valid and responsive to the clinical change that occurs over time. These properties are an attempt to closely define the subjective information we usually record, in a more robust (reliable) manner. These are discussed in detail in Section 2. A useful model is provided by Greenhalgh et al (1998). This is in the form of a checklist, see Table 3.2. This is the model used to evaluate OMs in Section 3.

Table 3.2 Evaluating an outcome measure for use in your practice

Evaluation	Questions to ask
Aim of the outcome measure *Is there information about why and how the measure was developed?* *How is it scored?*	What does the instrument plan to measure and was it originally designed for that purpose?
Content	**Describe the outcome measure**
User-centredness *Whose perspective does it capture?* *What domains are covered?* *What is the method of administration?*	Does the measure capture outcomes that are required by various users? Are the outcomes meaningful to the patient/client, the healthcare professional, a carer, the service provider or commissioner? Is the measure an observation of performance, a measure of opinions/attitudes or a self-reported measure of impact or performance? How does the scoring relate to the raw opinion or performance? Are there any distortions or biases present in the way the information is captured?
Measurement properties *What evidence is there about its reliability with this population?* *What evidence is there about its validity with this population?* *Is there information about how responsive to meaningful clinical change it is?*	Validity, reliability and measuring change – see Section 2.
Feasibility *Is there training required* *Lots of equipment* *Cost?*	How feasible is this OM to use in your clinical practice? Will the OM yield good quality data? Is the data easy to analyse and will reports be meaningful to both patients/clients and other interested parties? Is there a cost associated with its use?
Utility *How acceptable is it for you, for your patients?*	Will gathering this information be valuable to the patient/client? Will it be used in clinical decision-making? Does it provide unique information not available elsewhere? Will it capture the impact of a service?

Adapted from Greenhalgh et al 1998: 342.

Summary

There are many outcome measures available to help physiotherapists collect information about the outcome of their intervention. Choosing and using a measure is a skill that needs to be developed as much as any other professional skill, which will take time. It is vital that clinicians choose measures which relate to the aims of their intervention. Before choosing the measure, clinicians must appraise the quality of the measure. This involves making decisions based on published information about the measure, and considering its value and acceptability to patients in clinical practice.

Once a measure has been found, chosen and agreed for use, the most important part of evaluation starts: analysing the results and using them for the chosen purpose.

References

Binkley JM, Stratford PW, Lott SA, et al: The lower extremity functional scale: scale development, measurement properties, and clinical application, *Phys Ther* 79(4):371–383, 1999.

Cella DF, Dineen K, Arnason B, et al: Validation of the functional assessment of multiple sclerosis quality of life instrument, *Neurology* 47(1):29–39, 1996.

Clark M, Bond M: The Adelaide activities profile: a measure of lifestyle activities of elderly people aging, *Clin Exp Res* 7:174–184, 1995.

ER-WCPT: *European core standards of physiotherapy practice*, 2002, European Region of the World Confederation for Physical Therapy Online. Available: www.physio-europe.org/index.php?action=19. Accessed June 19, 2009.

Feinstein AR: The theory and evaluation on sensibility. In Feinstein AR, editor: *Clinimetrics*, New York, 1987, Yale University Press, pp 141–166.

Greenhalgh J, Long AF, Brettle AJ, et al: Reviewing and selecting outcome measures for use in routine practice, *J Eval Clin Pract* 4(4):339–350, 1998.

Grise MC, Gauthier-Gagnon C, Martineau GG: Prosthetic profile of people with lower extremity amputation: conception and design of a follow-up questionnaire, *Arch Phys Med Rehabil* 74(8):862–870, 1993.

Holden MK, Gill KM, Magliozzi MR, et al: Clinical gait assessment in the neurologically impaired: reliability and meaningfulness, *Phys Ther* 64:35–40, 1994.

IHW: *DASH outcome measure*, 2009, Institute for Health and Work. Online. Available: www.iwh.on.ca/dash-outcome-measure. Accessed June 19, 2009.

Le Roux AA: TELER: the concept, *Physiotherapy* 79(11):755–758, 1993.

Meenan RF, Gertman PM, Mason JH: Measuring health status in arthritis. The arthritis impact measurement scales, *Arthritis Rheum* 23(2):146–152, 1980.

Roos EM, Roos HP, Lohmander LS, et al: Knee injury and osteoarthritis outcome score (KOOS) Development of a self administered outcome measure, *J Orthop Sports Phys Ther* 78(2):88–96, 1998.

Smets EM, Garsen B, Bonke B, et al: The Multidimensional Fatigue Inventory (MFI): psychometric qualities of an instrument to assess fatigue, *J Psychosom Res* 39(3):315–325, 1995.

WCPT: *Draft position statement – physical therapy record keeping, storage and retrieval*, 2009, World Confederation for Physical Therapy. Online. Available: www.wcpt.org/node/29436. Accessed June 19, 2009.

Section 2

Measurement properties

This section considers the 'qualifications' of outcome measurements. These qualifications or measurement properties are often also referred to as the psycho-metric properties of measurements. They are often considered under the headings of reliability and validity. Reliability tells us how much error may exist within the measurement process and validity describes the attributes of the measurement, e.g. what it is similar to, what it contains, what patients/clients it can be used with. In addition, another property is the ability of the measurement to capture change in status over time. Two terms are used frequently: sensitivity and responsiveness. There is ongoing debate on the subject of sensitivity versus responsiveness and which of the two terms to use (Fritz 1999, Stratford et al 1999, Finch et al 2002). Kirshner & Guyatt (1985) first referred to 'responsiveness' as the power of the test to detect clinically relevant change. More recently, the two terms have been further defined by Liang (1995) as:

- Sensitivity: the ability to measure any change in a state
- Responsiveness: the ability to measure clinically meaningful or important change.

The author adds that responsiveness implies that the change is noticeable to the patient or the healthcare professional completed the measurement and may allow the person to perform a functional task more efficiently or with less pain or difficulty (Liang 2000). It is the term 'responsiveness' that is widely used in physiotherapy literature (Wright et al 1998, Stratford et al 1996, Hammond 2000, Finch et al 2002) and as such it will be used throughout this text.

There is also unresolved debate in the literature about where the ability of an instrument to measure change falls in the domains of measurement proper-ties. Some authors suggest that the responsiveness or sensitivity to change of an instrument is a separate measurement property and others believe it is part of the art–science continuum of activities that is incorporated in the investigation and evaluation of construct validity (Stratford et al 1996, Hays & Hadorn 1992, Guyatt et al 1987). Guyatt et al (1987) support the thesis that measurement respon-siveness/sensitivity is a property separate to validity and reliability, since it is possible to have a measure that is reliable but not responsive, responsive but not valid and unreliable but yet responsive. Hays & Hadorn (1992) respond to the thesis of Guyatt et al (1987) and suggest that while all of these situa-tions are indeed possible, the artificial distinction between responsiveness/sensitivity may arise from the desire to decide whether measurement instru-ments are either valid or not. The authors suggest that validity is in fact an ongoing iterative process and degrees of validity exist. Stratford et al (1996), in a paper describing the various methods that may be employed to establish measurement sensitivity/responsiveness and the analytical methods that may be employed, opts for including sensitivity/responsiveness as one component of validity. Cole et al (1995) note that for many outcome measures used by physiotherapists, a full examination of measurement properties has not been completed, and Liang (1995) note that sensitivity/responsiveness has had the least study. To a certain extent, where sensitivity/responsiveness is placed may be irrelevant as long as the property is examined and for the purposes of clarity in this book, it is presented separately from reliability and validity.

Chapter outlines

The following chapters introduce the concepts of:
- Reliability: Chapter 4
- Validity: Chapter 5
- Measuring change: Chapter 6.

Each chapter begins with a description of the measurement property and its sub-components, where relevant. Examples of the how these properties are evaluated and reported are provided as well as the various statistical tests that may be reported.

Reliability: error in measurement

4

CHAPTER CONTENTS

Introduction

Reliability tells us about the error that may exist in an outcome measure. It is commonly reported as inter-rater reliability and intra-rater reliability; this is informative but perhaps not immediately accessible for use in day-to-day clinical decision-making. In addition, another way to estimate reliability is to calculate the standard error of the measure which can then be used to calculate the minimal detectable change (MDC) of a measure; this is reported in the units of the outcome measure. MDC tells us how much change must happen for us to be sure it is true change and not simply measurement error.

Chapter outline

This chapter defines reliability and its component parts. It explores ways of establishing reliability and how it can be reported using descriptive and statistical methods.

What is reliability?

The measurement property of reliability refers to the degree to which an outcome measurement (OM) is free of random (McDowell 2006). Each observed score on an OM is the composite of the true score and random error. Random errors may occur during any part of the measuring process and may be a product of inattention, fatigue or inaccuracy. There are a variety of potential sources of error when using measurement instruments or outcome measurements. Other types of error, e.g. as a result of unclear instructions or interpretation of scores are normally considered during the design and development of the instrument (see Ch. 5). Rothstein (2001) suggested that reliability 'is not an all-or-none phenomenon, but rather it lies along a continuum'. Interpreting the ways in which reliability has been tested when an OM is being developed and considering the degree of reported error will be very important if the OM is used in practice.

Describing reliability

Reliability has been described as relative and absolute (Finch et al 2002). Absolute reliability is expressed as the standard error of the measurement (SEM) and is

DOI: 10.1016/B978-0-443-06915-4.00004-8

expressed in terms of the actual unit of the original instrument (Stratford 2004). This is probably of more use to the clinician on a day-to day basis than relative reliability. The SEM can be used to generate the minimal detectable change (MDC), which is the minimal amount of change in the score of an instrument that must occur in an individual in order to be sure that the change in score is not simply attributable to measurement error (Stratford et al 1996a, Stratford & Goldsmith 1997). MDC values are reported at 90% and 95% confidence levels. Estimating the MDC requires that a group of subjects are measured at two points, close enough to one another so that no change in performance is expected (Box 4.1).

The relative reliability of an instrument is often reported in three ways, inter-rater reliability, intra-rater reliability and internal consistency. Inter-rater reliability requires the same group of subjects to be measured at the same time by different observers. Intra-rater reliability considers the same subjects, the same rater and measurements taken at different time points. Internal consistency studies investigate the measurements of subjects in parallel (Finch et al 2002).

In evaluating the reliability of the Elderly Mobility Scale (EMS), Smith (1994) measured the performance of 15 older people. The two raters performed the measurements independently. Neither internal consistency nor intra-rater reliability was reported in the paper. A later study on the EMS considered inter-rater reliability using a similar method (Prosser & Canby 1997). Berg et al (1989) reported the inter- and intra-rater reliabilities in addition to the internal consistency of the Berg Balance Scale in the first paper published on the instrument. Five raters reviewed a videotaped performance of 14 subjects and the results of their scoring were compared. One week later, four of the raters reviewed the videotapes and re-scored the subjects, with a view

to considering the intra-rater reliability. The Postural Assessment Scale for Stroke Patients (PASS) is a scale for measuring the postural abilities in people with stroke. Similar methods were employed by Benaim et al (1999) to establish inter-rater reliability, i.e. two different raters reviewing 12 subjects with stroke and intra-rater reliability, i.e. one rater reviewed the same subjects 3 days later. It can be seen that while these methods seem similar, there are different potential sources of error within each of the designs. In the review of the BBS, all of the raters viewed the same subject, at the same time, on videotape. For the PASS study, the raters viewed the subjects separately but on the same day and this method was employed in the EMS studies. In the BBS study, the only source of error is the raters but in the other studies, there is an additional potential source of error and that is the patient/client error.

How are studies of reliability analysed?

The choice of method of analysis of reliability studies depends on the type of data (Box 4.2) generated by the OM, i.e. nominal, ordinal or interval/ratio.

Percentage agreement and kappa coefficients

Identifying the level of agreement between raters can be used as a simple and effective way of illustrating the level of agreement but it does not take into consideration the proportion of agreement that is

Box 4.2

Types of data

Nominal or categorical information is when numbers are assigned to categories, e.g.
   1 = male, 3 = female.
   Ordinal data also employs numbers and many rehabilitation outcome measures have ordinal outputs. The numbers represent changes in performance but are not absolute. For example, a score of 20/56 on the Berg Balance Scale does not mean the performance is half that of a score of 40/56.
   Interval scales have units of change that are equivalent to one another, e.g. temperature. Ratio scales also have constant unit changes but have a meaningful zero (0), e.g. time and range of motion.

Box 4.1

Minimal detectable change in the Berg Balance Scale

Stevenson (2001) evaluated the minimal detectable change of the Berg Balance Scale in people with stroke. To be sure that real change has occurred in balance in people with stroke who can mobilize independently or with standby assistance, their performance must change >5 points between testing times. If the patient requires assistance, then the Berg Balance Scale (BBS) must change >7 points for the change to be real change.

attributable simply to chance (Streiner & Norman 1989). The kappa coefficient (κ) corrects for chance agreement by calculating the extent of agreement that could exist between raters by chance. The weighted kappa coefficient (κw) (Cohen 1968) extends this concept and allows for partial agreement between raters, e.g. a difference of 1 in the scores between raters or times of rating is not considered to be a difference.

Gregson et al (2000) used % agreement and κw when investigating the Modified Ashworth Scale in people with stroke. Table 4.1 outlines some of their results for intra-rater reliability.

How do we interpret these results? Percentage agreement for rater A between measurements taken at time 1 and time 2 ranged from 52–79% depending on the joint being tested, the range for rater B, a research physiotherapist, were similar: 50–71%. Interpreting the κw according to Brennan & Silman (1992), suggests that the level of agreement noted varied from 'moderate' to 'very good'. Interestingly, certain items in a scale may demonstrate more or less agreement than others. In evaluating the intra-rater reliability of the PASS, Benaim et al (1999) report a κ coefficient of 0.45 for 'sitting without support' and 1 for 'standing on the paretic leg'. Kappa values of 0.61–0.8 indicate substantial agreement and >0.8 suggest almost perfect agreement (Landis & Koch 1977).

Table 4.1 Percentage agreement and κw for the modified Ashworth Scale

MAS – Joint	Rater[a]	Agreement between time 1 and time 2 (%)	κw	What the κw means
Elbow	A	72	0.77	Good
Wrist	A	59	0.88	Very good
Knee	A	79	0.94	Very good
Ankle	A	52	0.64	Good
Elbow	B	62	0.83	Very good
Wrist	B	71	0.80	Good
Knee	B	50	0.77	Good
Ankle	B	73	0.59	Moderate

[a]A, Medical specialist registrar; B, Research physiotherapist.
From Gregson et al (2000).

Intra-class correlation

For measurements that generate continuous data, analysis of variance (ANOVA) can be employed and a resulting intra-class correlation is reported (Deyo & Centor 1986, Streiner & Norman 1989, Finch et al 2002, McDowell 2006). The intra-class correlation coefficient (ICC) is an indication of the variance due to error. This is calculated using different contributory sources of variance. In a study where two observers rate a number of subjects, there will be variance between and within subjects and observers and random error. Six different forms of ICC are described by Shrout and Fleiss (1979) for inter-rater reliability and each depends on the design of the study and the later use of the instrument whose reliability is being tested. It is important that the type of ICC used is reported as well as the reasons why it was chosen. Pomeroy and Tallis (2000) investigated the reliability of using a 100 mm visual analogue scale (VAS) for testing tone. The lower end of the scale represented 'lowest tone possible' and the highest end was 'highest tone possible'. Tone was tested by 6 physiotherapists in a sample of healthy people and those with chronic stroke and the ICC reported was 0.451 for knee extensor tone and 0.595 for elbow extensor tone. Since the closer to 1 the ICC is, the more reliable the OM, these results suggest that the VAS method employed to evaluate tone was not reliable. Reid et al (2007) used the ICC (2,1) to evaluate 'hop testing' following anterior cruciate ligament repair and report ICCs ranging from 0.82 to 0.93 and this test was also employed by De Wit et al (2007) when investigating the reliability of a list to define the content of individual physiotherapy and occupational therapy sessions for people with stroke, reporting ICCs of 0.71–1. Despite the recommendation by McDowell (2006) and Rankin & Stokes (1998), only one of these studies described the exact ICC employed.

Bland and Altman method

Bland and Altman (1995) report an accurate method of assessing the degree of error between sets of data either between raters or at different points in time, over the full range of reported scores. If two raters generate two sets of scores, we can plot the mean of the sets of scores against the differences of the two sets of scores and it is possible to consider if error changes over the range of the scale. Figure 4.1 illustrates the mean versus the difference for the Berg

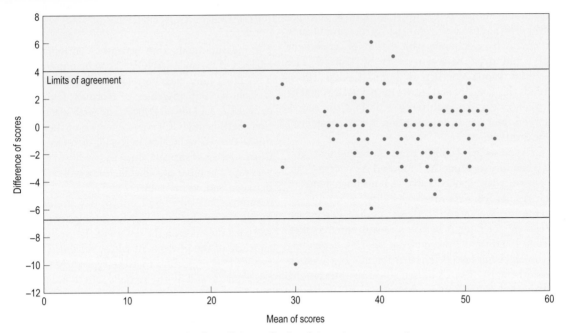

Figure 4.1 • Bland and Altman plot for Berg Balance Scale – intra-rater agreement.

Balance Scale measured at two different points in time (intra-rater reliability).

The mean of the differences (−0.64) and the standard deviation (SD) of the differences (2.47) is then calculated. The 95% limits of agreement can then be calculated: the mean of the differences ± 1.96 × SD of the differences (−5.5 to 4.2 in this example). In this Figure 4.1, it can be seen that almost all the points within the limits of agreement, suggesting a high level of agreement. This method is reported by Benaim et al (1999) and Stokes et al (1998) when analysing the inter- and intra-rater reliabilities of rehabilitation outcome measures.

Internal consistency

A further method of analysing a measurement instrument for reliability is termed internal consistency. This is also a measure of the homogeneity of the instrument. In essence, the relationship between the items and their relationship with the overall score is considered. The higher the relationship between the individual items, the easier it would be to create two similar versions that are reliable, thus improving test–re-test reliability. Nevertheless, inter-item correlation should not be too strong because it may negate the need to retain strongly related items. All the items should relate to the total score because this supports the construct that one theme or domain is being

measured, albeit through the contributory components. Internal consistency may be reported through the expression of inter-item correlations, using the Pearson-product moment correlation coefficient (PPMCC) to illustrate the level of association between the items (Streiner & Norman 1989). When comparing individual items to the overall score, the latter should exclude the individual item to which it is being compared. The most common statistical expression of internal consistency is Cronbach's alpha (α) (Streiner & Norman 1989, Finch et al 2002, McDowell 2006). Bland & Altman (1997) suggest that for scales that will be used to compare two groups in research studies, alpha can be less than ones for use with individuals in clinical practice. For the latter, the minimum α is 0.90. Berg et al (1989) reported a Cronbach's α of 0.96 for the BBS with inter-item correlations ranging from 0.71–0.89. Benaim et al (1999) reported a Cronbach's α of 0.95 for PASS; the authors did not report inter-item correlation coefficients.

Error reported in the units of outcome measure – standard error of the measurement

The standard error of the measurement (SEM) can be calculated in a number of ways (Stratford 2004) and by providing this additional information in reliability studies may provide more meaningful

Table 4.2 Methods to calculate the SEM

Method	Design	Output	SEM
Method 1	Testing at two time points, with both sets of data having equal variance (SD)	Standard deviation (SD) and Pearson's correlation coefficient (r)	$s\sqrt{1-r}$
Method 2A	Testing at two time points	One-way ANOVA to calculate relative reliability. Use Mean Squares for within subjects from ANOVA table	$\sqrt{MSW}$
Method 2B	Testing at two time points but with a randomized block format	One-way ANOVA to calculate relative reliability. Use Mean Squares error term from ANOVA table	$\sqrt{MSE}$
Method 3	Testing at two time points	Estimate the SD of the difference scores	$SD/\sqrt{2}$

From Stratford (2004). $\sqrt{}$, square root.

data to physiotherapists. Table 4.2 illustrates the methods that may be used to calculate the SEM (Stratford 2004).

Its interpretation is that there is a 68% chance that a true score will fall within ± 1 SEM of the observed score. To ascertain 95% confidence levels the SEM is multiplied by 1.96. In order to calculate the MDC at this level, the calculation is as follows:

$$\text{SEM} \times 1.96 \times \sqrt{2}$$

The incorporation of the $\sqrt{2}$ allows for the fact that error may also occur as a result of two measuring episodes. Although the SEM is reported to be relatively constant across all levels of a population's ability, except extremes, SEMs are reported for a variety of different initial scores (Stratford et al 1996a, 1998).The Neck Disability Index (NDI) is an outcome measure used to assess the disability of patients with neck pain, its MDC_{90} is reported as 5 points (Stratford et al 1999). The MDC_{95} and MDC_{90} for the Berg Balance Scale are reported as 6.9 and 5.8 points, respectively (Stevenson 2001). In this study, Stevenson demonstrates that in a group of subjects with stroke who were still receiving in-patient rehabilitation, the MDC_{95} may vary depending on functional status from 6.0 points in subjects who require standby assistance to 8.1 in those who require assistance. In older people having rehabilitation, a change of 4 points in the BBS is needed to be 95% confident that true change has occurred if a patient scores within 45–56 initially; 5 points if they score within 35–44; 7 points if they score within 25–34; and finally 5 points if their initial score is within 0–24 on the BBS (Donoghue et al 2009). Conditional MDC_{90} of 4–5 points is reported for the Roland Morris Questionnaire, since the authors (Stratford et al 1996b) note that this applies only to subjects with initial scores of between 4 and 20 on the scale.

What not to use or to interpret with caution

The Pearson-product moment correlation coefficient (PPMCC) is frequently cited in support of the reliability of an instrument. Nonetheless, it not an accurate representation of the level of agreement between raters or within a rater and may exaggerate reliability (Bland & Altman 1986, McDowell 2006). The PPMCC reflects the degree to which two sets of continuous data have a liner relationship so it represents the association between data but not the agreement between it. Thus, the two sets of data in Table 4.3

Table 4.3 Reliability datasets

Subject	Dataset 1	Dataset 2
1	10	20
2	12	22
3	14	24
4	22	32
5	32	42
6	34	44
7	35	45
8	28	38
9	23	33
10	14	24

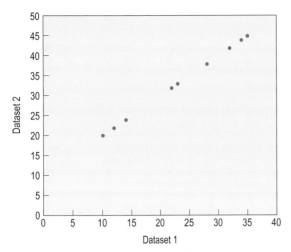

Figure 4.2 • Scatterplots of data in Table 4.3.

indeed, if it reflects two raters measuring the same subject at the same time, despite reporting a very high PPMCC, there is no agreement between the raters. Hence, when interpreting the results of reliability studies on measurement instruments, the PPMCC should be interpreted with caution. The same applies when the Spearman Rank correlation coefficient is reported for other types of data.

Summary

Reliability gives us an indication of the extent to which error may exist in the OMs we use in clinical practice. We need to understand this so that we can evaluate whether the results we get when we measure a patient or client's performance may have been influenced by some possibility of error. There are various ways of investigating reliability and it is reported using different descriptive and statistical methods. Table 4.4 summarizes the various ways of investigating and reporting reliability.

yield the scatterplot in Figure 4.2 and a PPMCC of 1.0. If this represents the same rater measuring the same subjects at different times (but with no anticipated changes in the subjects' scores), or

Table 4.4 Measurement properties and what how they inform choice and decision-making

Measurement property	Component of property	Definition	What does it tell us?	Statistical expressions reported in the literature	For more information and examples
Reliability	Relative – inter- and intra-	The agreement between raters or between two points in time	An indication of the amount of random error that exists in the SOM	Correlation coefficients (interpret with caution), Bland & Altman method, % agreement, kappa and weighted kappa coefficients, intra-class correlation coefficients	Gregson et al (2000) Mao et al (2002) Pomeroy & Tallis (2000) Stokes & Rankin (1998)
	Absolute reliability	An indication of reliability expressed in the units of the original measurement	The amount of change that needs to take place to me more that measurement error	Minimal detectable change – both 90% and 95% confidence levels can be expressed	Stevenson (2001) Stratford (2004)
	Internal consistency	Measurements taken at one point in time, an indication of the homogeneity of the SOM	Relationship between the individual items in the SOM and the overall score	Cronbach's alpha	Berg et al (1989) Benaim et al (1999)

References

Benaim C, Perennou DA, Villy J, et al: Validation of a standardised assessment of postural control in stroke patients, *Stroke* 30:1862–1868, 1999.

Berg KO, Wood-Dauphinee SL, Williams JI, et al: Measuring balance in the elderly: preliminary development of an instrument, *Physiother Can* 41:304–311, 1989.

Bland JM, Altman DG: Statistical methods for assessing agreement between two methods of clinical measurement, *Lancet* 1:07–310, 1986.

Bland JM, Altman DG: Comparing methods measurement: why plotting difference against standard method is misleading, *Lancet* 346:1085–1087, 1997.

Bland JM, Altman DG: Statistics notes Cronbach's alpha, *BMJ* 314:572, 1995.

Brennan P, Silman A: Statistical methods for assessing observer variability in clinical measures, *BMJ* 304: 1941–1944, 1992.

Cole B, Finch E, Gowland C, et al: Basmajian J, editor: *Physical rehabilitation outcome measures*, Baltimore, 1995, Williams and Wilkins.

Cohen J: Weighted kappa: nominal scale agreement with provision for scaled disagreement or partial credit, *Psychol Bull* 70:213–220, 1968.

De Wit L, Kamsteegt H, Yadav B, et al: Defining the content of individual physiotherapy and occupational therapy sessions for stroke patients in an inpatient rehabilitation setting. Development, validation and inter-rater reliability of a scoring list, *Clin Rehabil* 21(5):450–460, 2007.

Deyo RA, Centor RM: Assessing the responsiveness of functional scales to clinical change: an analogy to diagnostic test performance, *J Chronic Dis* 39:897–906, 1986.

Donoghue D, Physiotherapy Research and Older People (PROP) group, Stokes EK: How much change is true change? The minimum detectable change of the Berg Balance Scale in elderly people, *J Rehabil Med* 41 (5):343–346, 2009.

Finch E, Brooks D, Stratford P, et al: *Physical rehabilitation outcome measures – A guide to enhanced clinical decision making*, ed 2, Ontario, 2002, BC Decker.

Fritz JM: Sensitivity to change (letter), *Phys Ther* 79(4):420–421, 1999.

Gregson JM, Leathley MJ, Moore AP, et al: Reliability of measurements of muscle tine and muscle power in stroke patients, *Age Ageing* 29:223–228, 2000.

Guyatt G, Walter S, Norman G: Measuring changes over time: the usefulness of evaluative instruments, *J Chronic Dis* 40:171–178, 1987.

Hammond R: Evaluation of physiotherapy by measuring the outcome, *Physiotherapy* 86(4): 170–172, 2000.

Hays RD, Hadorn D: Responsiveness to change: an aspect of validity, not a separate dimension, *Qual Life Res* 1:73–75, 1992.

Kirshner B, Guyatt G: A methodological framework for assessing health indices, *J Chronic Dis* 38(1):27–36, 1985.

Landis JR, Koch GG: The measurement of observer agreement for categorical data, *Biometrics* 33:159–174, 1977.

Liang MH: Longitudinal construct validity: establishment of clinical meaning in patient evaluation instruments, Med Care 38 Suppl 11: II-89–90, 2000.

Liang MH: Evaluating measurement responsiveness, *J Rheumatol* 22:1191–1192, 1995.

Mao HF, Hseuh IP, Tang PF, et al: Analysis and comparison of the psychometric properties of three balance measures for stroke patients, *Stroke* 33:1022–1027, 2002.

McDowell I: *Measuring Health, A guide to Rating Scales and Questionnaires*, ed 2, New York, 2006, Oxford University Press.

Pomeroy V, Tallis R: Physical therapy to improve movement performance and functional ability post stroke. Part 1: existing evidence, *Rev Clin Gerontol* 10:261–290, 2000.

Prosser L, Canby A: Further validation of the Elderly Mobility Scale for measurement of mobility of hospitalised elderly, *Clin Rehabil* 11:338–343, 1997.

Rankin G, Stokes M: Reliability of assessment tools in rehabilitation: an illustration of appropriate statistical analyses, *Clin Rehabil* 12:187–199, 1998.

Reid A, Birmingham TB, Stratford PW: Hop testing provides a reliable and valid outcome measure during rehabilitation after anterior cruciate ligament reconstruction, *Phys Ther* 87 (3):337–350, 2007.

Rothstein J: Sick and tired of reliability. Editor's note, *Phys Ther* 81 (2):774–776, 2001.

Shrout PE, Fleiss JL: Intraclass correlations: uses in assessing rater reliability, *Psychol Bull* 86 (2):420–428, 1979.

Smith R: Validation and reliability of the Elderly Mobility Scale, *Physiotherapy* 80(11):744–747, 1994.

Stevenson TJ: Detecting change in patients with stroke using the Berg Balance Scale, *Aust J Physiother* 47:29–38, 2001.

Stokes EK, Finn AM, Walsh JB, et al: The 'Balance-Meter': investigation of an apparatus to measure postural sway, *Health Care in Later Life* 3 (3):215–225, 1998.

Stratford PW, Goldsmith CH: Use of the standard error as a reliability index of interest: an applied example using elbow flexor strength data, *Phys Ther* 77(7):745–750, 1997.

Stratford PW, Binkley JM, Riddle DL: Health status measures and analytic methods for assessing change scores, *Phys Ther* 76(10):1109–1123, 1996a.

Stratford PW, Binkley J, Soloman P, et al: Defining the minimal detectable change for the Roland-Morris Questionnaire, *Phys Ther* 76 (4):350–368, 1996b.

Stratford PW, Binkley J, Riddle D, et al: Sensitivity to change of the Roland-Morris Back Pain Questionnaire: Part 1, *Phys Ther* 78(11):1186–1195, 1998.

Stratford PW, Riddle DL, Binkley JM, et al: Using the Neck Disability Index to make decisions concerning individual patients, *Physiother Can* Spring, 107–112, 119, 1999.

Stratford PW: Getting more from the literature: estimating the standard error of the measurement from reliability studies, *Physiother Can* 56 (1):27–30, 2004.

Streiner DL, Norman GR: *Health Measurement Scales, A practical guide to their development and use*, Oxford, 1989, Oxford University Press.

Wright J, Cross J, Lamb S: Physiotherapy outcome measures for rehabilitation of elderly people. Responsiveness to change of the Rivermead Mobility Index and Barthel Index, Physiotherapy 84(5):216–221, 1998.

Validity

CHAPTER CONTENTS

Introduction

The validity of outcome measures is investigated and reported in many ways. The traditional methods are being enhanced with the use of different statistical techniques, such as Rasch analysis. In the initial stages of development, the face and content validity should be reported. This tells us what work the designers carried out in order to decide what items to include in the outcome measure. The results of their research are often reported in descriptive terms, however some statistical tests can also be used such as factor analysis.

Validity also compares relationships, e.g. the relationship that exists between the new outcome measure and a nominated *gold standard* measure or an exploration of the extent to which a new outcome measure relates to other scales and outcome measures at this point in time or in the future. We may expect some groups of patients/client to perform better than others or indeed individuals, who do not have a particular condition to score better than those who have the condition. If this is the case, some evaluation may be made about how the new outcome measure discriminates between groups of people.

The evaluation of the validity of an outcome measure may result in changes to the outcome measure and may yield a new version of the original measure. The later iterations may be similar in length to the original but with different scoring or instructions, or may be shortened for ease of use. In addition, an outcome measure which was originally designed for use with one patient/client group may be validated for use with a different group or a different method e.g. in person versus telephone interview. Hence, the process of validation is iterative and organic and responsive to new calls placed on the outcome measure in clinical practice.

Chapter outline

This chapter discusses ways of establishing if an outcome measure (OM) is valid. The various types of validity are described, how they can be reported and their relevance to clinical practice.

DOI: 10.1016/B978-0-443-06915-4.00005-X

The description and methodology of validity

Face, content, criterion, construct, convergent . . . the list is endless of terms used when describing the validity. The purpose of this chapter is to explain the various different ways of evaluation validity and how they may be reported in the literature. Thereafter, we try to help the reader understand the relevance of the reportage for clinical practice and decision-making.

Face and content validity

Face validity is, as the name suggests, a question of whether on the face or surface of the outcome measurement (OM) it measures what it intends to measure. If the face validity is good, then it is more likely to be acceptable to users. If items seem irrelevant to their practice, it is possible they will simply be omitted (Streiner & Norman 1989).

Streiner and Norman (1989) suggest that face validity and content validity are generally defined within the sphere of subjective professional consensus or require an explicit process which includes establishing the theoretical framework of the measure, research and expert opinion based on clinical observation. These inform which items should be considered for inclusion, before the OM is submitted for further measurement testing.

If an instrument contains within it a number of domains that represent a sample of the total population of domains (most likely theoretical) that could be included, content validity considers how adequate the sample of domains is, with regard to the expected functionality of the instrument. If an instrument aims to measure functional mobility in older people, the content validity of the OM is a measure of how well the constituent parts reflect the aim of the instrument, which should be clearly stated in the design phase (McDowell 2006).

According to Feinstein (1987), content validity requires digging deeper than face validity. It requires consideration of not simply the components that are included and their suitability but also important omissions. He also considers the output of the domains that constitute the instrument, scaling and weighting. The above descriptions of face and content validity are supported throughout the literature on measurement properties (Green 1981, Bush 2000, Finch et al 2002).

In the descriptions of the development of instruments, it is often not explicitly stated how face and content validity have been considered (Reuben & Siu 1990, Di Fabio & Seay 1997). Nonetheless, in some cases, brief descriptions are given, e.g. in the development of the Elderly Mobility Scale, which employed discussion with physiotherapists, and a literature review (Smith 1994). Tinetti (1986) describes the process as a review of 'previous work by bioengineers, orthopedists, neurologists, rheumatologists, and physical therapists to identify what observations should be included'. Platt et al (1998) used a panel of physiotherapists in the development of the Physiotherapy Functional Mobility Profile. Berg et al (1989), in the preliminary development of the eponymous balance scale, considered face and content validity in three phases. Using both professional samples (physiotherapists, nurses, physicians and occupational therapists) and patient samples (older people with an impairment of balance), groups of items were identified as being important for inclusion in the scale. The next phase asked the healthcare professionals to rank the importance of the items and asked the patients to rate their sense of unsteadiness when performing the activities. The third iteration of the scale was further tested on patients and their responses were compared with the scores they achieved on the scale. The healthcare professionals were asked to view videotapes of patients performing the items in the scale and asked to identify which components were essential for inclusion and which were extraneous. The final iteration of the scale was tested for reliability using five physiotherapists. It resulted in the production of a 14-item instrument, which is scored on a 5-point ordinal scale. Box 5.1 illustrates how this can help us in clinical practice.

Criterion validity

Following the consideration of face and content validity, more formal evaluation of validity is conducted. Criterion validity considers the performance

---

Box 5.1

What does this tell us for clinical practice?

Take a look at an outcome measure you currently use or are planning to use and see how the designers planned its construction. Were users involved in the design? Do you think the components are meaningful to you? Do your patients/clients think they are relevant to them?

or accuracy (Feinstein 1987) of the new instrument by comparing it to a *gold standard*. The level of agreement between the two sets of measurements is then examined, using an 'appropriate indicator of agreement' (McDowell 2006); since this is often a correlational comparison, criterion validity may also be referred to as correlational validity.

The *gold standard* may often be a more expensive or time-consuming version of the new OM, e.g. in designing a portable device for measuring strength, the new OM might be compared with an isokinetic dynamometer. A new field test of fitness or exercise tolerance would be compared with a laboratory test such as VO$_2$max.

There is a timing component associated with this type of validity – it can be either concurrent or predictive:

- Concurrent validity is how the new instrument compares with the *gold standard* at a given point in time
- Predictive validity refers to its relationship to an assessment in the future.

In describing how criterion validity is assessed, Streiner and Norman (1989) pose the following question: If a good criterion measure exists, why create another instrument? That the new instrument is less expensive, less invasive or carries less risk, are the main reasons for creating a new means of measurement. The consideration of criterion validity becomes less absolute when a *gold standard* does not exist. This is often the case for rehabilitation measures. Nevertheless, criterion validity may still be assessed by substituting other well known and accepted OMs as a substitute for the *gold standard*. Table 5.1 illustrates a variety of ways the criterion validity has been established for a sample of physiotherapy scales.

What do the statistics tell us?

The output of criterion validity and convergent validity (an aspect of construct validity discussed later) will be validity coefficients. These are products of correlating the scores obtained on the new instrument with a *gold standard* or with existing measurements of similar domains. The validity coefficients can range from -1 to $+1$.

- *Pearson-product moment correlation (PPMCC)* – consideration of the linear relationship between OM where the OM measures interval or ratio data, e.g. time, range of motion in degrees. If the data from two sets of measurements are plotted against one another, the PPMCC illustrates the closeness of the points to a straight line: $+1$ or -1 indicating a string relationship, and 0 indicating no relationship at all
- *Spearman's rank order correlation*. When x and y are not linearly related, but show a consistently increasing or decreasing trend in rank, a non-parametric correlation such as Spearman's (ρ) may be employed. It assumes that the data are ordinal, e.g. many of the OMs in rehabilitation
- *Kendall's rank order correlation (τ)*. This coefficient may be applied in cases where Spearman's rho is appropriate.
- *Phi coefficient (ψ)*. Used in the analysis of data which is dichotomous i.e. presence of absence of a disease.

Box 5.2 indicates how we might interpret these results for clinical practice.

Table 5.1 Examples of concurrent and predictive validity

Author	New scale	Validity	Compared with a cognate scale
Smith (1994)	Elderly Mobility Scale (EMS)	Concurrent	Barthel Index (BI) Functional Independence Measure (FIM)
Prosser & Canby (1997)			Barthel Index
Collen et al (1991)	Rivermead Mobility Index (RMI)	Concurrent	BI, Functional Ambulation Categories (FAC), gait speed, 6-min distance test (SMDT)
Benaim et al (1999)	Postural Assessment Scale for Stroke (PASS)	Concurrent and predictive	FIM-transfers, locomotion, total concurrent measure and at 90 days after stroke
Mao et al (2002)			BI, Berg Balance Scale (BBS)

Box 5.2

How we interpret these results for clinical practice

How good is the result? When the output of two outcome measurements is compared, a maximum possible correlation between them exists and this is the square root of the product of their respective reliabilities.

McDowell (2006) set out an example of how this might be used to inform a making a judgement about a result. If we were to compare two outcome measures, e.g. a field test of fitness (field fit) and a laboratory test of fitness (lab fit) and our result is 0.6, we need to know one other piece of information and that is the reliability coefficient for each test. Let us say they are 0.7 for field fit and 0.75 for lab fit. According to Helmstadter (1966) this should be considered

in light of the maximum possible coefficient of validity, which would be 0.72. So the result of 0.6 is very good.

However, we should also consider what strength of a relationship we might expect, given our clinical knowledge. From Table 5.2, it can be seen that the Berg Balance Scale has been compared with many other OMs. Some are laboratory tests and others are more functional but not necessarily with a focus on balance, e.g. Barthel Index.

Remember that when you compare 'like with like' you would expect a stronger relationship. Sometimes the coefficient is negative (−) and this means that a high score on one OM is related to a low score on the other OM.

Table 5.2 Reported coefficients of validity for the Berg Balance Scale

Author	Subjects	Validity co-efficient	Variable compared to BSS	Coefficient
Stevenson & Garland (1996)	24 subjects 8.4 ± 6.16 years post-stroke. 68.8 ± 7.72 years*	Pearson-product moment correlation coefficient (PPMCC)	Mean centre of pressure (COP) speed in quiet stance	−0.76
			Mean COP speed during arm flexion	−0.65
			Peak arm acceleration	−0.67
Wolf et al (1999)	28 subjects with stroke, 56.4 ± 13.8 years*, 162.5–190.5 months post-stroke	PPMCC	Functional reach	0.62
			Gait speed	0.63
Usuda et al (1998)	46 subjects with stroke, 69.3 ± 9.6 years*	Spearman's rank order coefficient (SRCC)	Barthel Index	0.84
			Brunnstrom's recovery stage	0.56
Shumway-Cook et al (1997)	44 community dwelling older people – faller 77.6 ± 5.4 years* and non-fallers, 74.6 ± 54 years*	SRCC	Use of assistive device	−0.53
			History of imbalance	−0.50
			Balance self-perceptions	0.76
			Dynamic Gait Index	0.67
Kokko et al (1997)	40 patients with Parkinson's disease, mean age 67 years, range 35–84 years	PPMCC	Relative gait velocity (height/speed for 10 m)	0.56
			Relative stride length	0.60
			Hand dexterity	0.56
			Functional Status Questionnaire	0.67
Piotrowski & Cole (1994)	60 older people volunteers – nursing home residents and community dwelling, 78 ± 6.88 years*	PPMCC	Falls efficacy scale	0.86
			Functional Assessment Inventory	0.86
			Self-paced walk test	0.73
Hsieh et al (2000)	38 subjects with stroke	SRCC	Rivermead Mobility Index	0.80
Nilsson et al (1998)	28 subjects, 3–8 weeks post-stroke, 55 ± 9.3 years*	SRCC	Step frequency over 10 m	−0.69
			Borg Category Scale	−0.73
			Functional Ambulation Category	0.63

*Mean age and standard deviation (years).

Predicting the future – how can we use OMs to predict future events?

Sensitivity and specificity, positive and negative predictive values, likelihood ratios

How good is an OM in predicting falls or the likelihood of a person returning to work? The ability of an OM in identifying correctly the presence of a disease/disorder/condition in an individual (sensitivity), but also its precision in correctly identifying that the disease/disorder/condition is not present (specificity), are considered as part of criterion validity.

Sensitivity and specificity are reported in percentages, which are generated as a result of a type of 2×2 table (see Table 5.3).

Sensitivity is calculated as $100\% \times (a/[a+c])$ and specificity as $100\% \times (d/[d+b])$. Using data from two studies on the Berg Balance Scale (BBS), Riddle and Stratford (1999) explore the sensitivity and specificity of this scale. The BBS is a scale that measures balance in older people. It is scored out of 56, with higher scores suggesting better balance. A single cut-off point of <45/56 has been utilized to identify people at risk of falling. Combining the data from the two previously published studies (Bogle Thorbahn & Newton 1996, Shumway-Cook et al 1997) and using the cut-off point of <45/56 to identify those at risk of falling, yielded a sensitivity of 64% and a specificity of 90%. This suggests that one of three fallers were missed by the BBS and that it is more accurate in identifying non-fallers, since only 10% of them were incorrectly identified. The authors note that

since sensitivity and specificity are not dependent on the prevalence of the disorder, the information can be applied to how useful the BBS will be when used with any group of older people with balance disorders.

Other ways of reporting the ability of an OM to be predictive are positive and negative predictive values (PPV and NPV). PPV is the proportion of subjects with a positive test result who have the condition of interest and the NPV being the proportion of subjects with a negative test result who do not have the condition. If a positive predictive value is near 100% it is more likely that the disease or condition being predicted by the test is actually present when the test is positive.

Box 5.3 suggests how we might interpret PPV and NPV results for clinical practice.

Whereas sensitivity considers the instrument and its ability to identify subjects or patients who have a disorder, positive predictive values (PPV) focus on the number of people correctly identified by the test as having the condition.

Likelihood ratios (LRs) combine sensitivity and specificity and give an indication of how much a particular score (or range of scores) on a outcome measure instrument or test will raise or lower the pre-test probability of a particular condition being present, e.g. falls risk, improvement in pain (Fritz et al 2000). In other words, how much better would you be at predicting a condition if you were to rely on your clinical judgement as well as scores on the outcome measure.

A simple review of therapy literature reveals a number of studies of outcome measures or clinical tests where the LRs were evaluated (Table 5.4). Some investigators wished to ascertain if certain scores on a measurement could predict whether patients/clients would return to work, others wished

Table 5.3 2×2 table

Result of test	Gold standard or criterion		Total
	Condition present	Condition absent	
Condition present	True positive (a)	False positive (b)	a+b
Condition absent	False negative (c)	True negative (d)	c+d
Total	a+c	b+d	

Box 5.3

How do we interpret PPV and NPV results for clinical practice?

Let us say that the OM you use is known to be able to predict if a patient/client will walk independently and a score of >7/10 suggests that the client/patient will walk independently. The OM has a PPV of 90%, so you can say that 9 out of 10 patients/clients who have a positive test result, i.e. score of greater >7/10 will be correctly predicted to walk independently.

Table 5.4 Likelihood ratios in therapy research

Author	Profile of participants	Predicted end-point	Measurement	Likelihood ratio (LR) (95% CI)	Pre-test probability	Post-test probability
Werneke & Hart (2004)	Acute work-related low back pain, 1 year after discharge (n = 171)	Return to work status	Pain pattern classification, time dependent, i.e. after intervention completed. Presence or absence of centralization of pain	+LR 3.82 (2.29–6.35) −LR 0.38 (0.2–0.75)	15%	25%
Fritz & George (2002)	Acute work-related low back pain (n = 78)	Persistent work restrictions	Work sub-scale of Fear Avoidance Beliefs (FAB) Questionnaire 0–42, higher = more FAB +LR >34/42 −LR <30/42	>34 +LR 3.33 (1.05–6.77) <30/42 −LR 0.08 (0.01–0.54)	29%	>34/42 (58%) <30/42 (3%)
Sutlive et al (2004)	Patello-femoral pain syndrome (n = 45)	Reduction in pain, i.e. >50% improvement on VAS	Forefoot valgus (FFV) ≥2° Passive great toe extension (PGTE) ≤78° Navicular drop (ND) <3 mm	FFV≥2° +LR 4.0 (0.7–21.9) PGTE +LR 4.0 (0.7–21.9) ND +LR 2.3 (1.3–4.3)	60%	Forefoot valgus (FFV) ≥2° (86%) Passive great toe extension (PGTE) ≤78° (86%) Navicular drop (ND) <3 mm (78%)
Fritz et al (2000)	Return-to-work within 4 weeks, following occupational acute low back pain (n = 69)	5 non-organic signs (NOSg) and 7 non-organic symptom descriptors (NOSymp) and non-organic index (NOI)	≥2 NOSg ≥3 NOSymp ≥3 NOI	≥2 NOSg −LR 0.75 (0.51–1.10) ≥3 NOSymp −LR 0.62 (0.40–0.96) ≥3 NOI −LR 0.59 (0.32–1.07)	33%	−NOSg (27%) −NOSymp (24%) −NOI (23%)

Study	Description	Measure	Value	Sensitivity	Specificity
Stratford et al (1998)	Investigation of test characteristics of Roland-Morris Questionnaire in subjects with low back pain of <6 weeks (n = 226)	Global rating of change in status, score of change = 5	Roland Morris Questionnaire (RMQ) change score of ≥5	4 (2.49–6.37)	63%	87%
Riddle et al (1998)	Investigation of test characteristics of Roland-Morris Questionnaire in subjects with low back pain (n = 143)	Chance of achieving treatment goals	Roland Morris Questionnaire (RMQ) important change score, for different initial (iRMQ) scores, e.g. 0–8, 9–16, 17–24	iRMQ 0–8 +LR 5.33 (1.47–20.4) iRMQ 9–16 +LR 3.7 (1.35–10.02) iRMQ 17–24 +LR 4.55 (1.33–15.28)	iRMQ 0–8 (78%) iRMQ 9–16 (72%) iRMQ 17–24 (57%)	iRMQ 0–8 (95%) iRMQ 9–16 (86%) iRMQ 17–24 (86%)
Abbott & Mercer (2003)	Patients with low back pain (new or also within previous 3 months) or those with persistent pain of at least 3 months duration (n = 12)	Presence of lumbar segmental hypomobility, defined using radiography	Active range of motion of lumbar spine (AROM) Abnormality of segmental motion during AROM (AbnROM) Passive accessory inter-vertebral movements (PAIVM) Passive physiological intervertebral movements (PPIVM)	AROM +LR 1.88 (0.57–6.8) −LR 0.42 (0.07–1.9) AbnROM +LR 3.6 (0.84–15.38) −LR 0.65 (0.28–1.06) PAIVM +LR 1.16 (0.44–2.03) −LR 0.71 (0.12–2.75) PPIVM +LR 3.86 (0.89–16.31) −LR 0.64 (0.28–1.04)	28%	+AROM signs (≈41%) +AbnROM signs (58%)* +PAIVM signs (≈30%) +PPIVM signs (≈60%) −AROM signs (14%) −AbnROM signs (≈20%) −PAIVM signs (≈22%) −PPIVM signs (≈20%)

41

to investigate if fear avoidance behaviour scores could predict how back pain restricted work behaviours. Using an active range of motion of the lumbar spine (AROM) was also considered as a predictor of the presence of lumbar segmental hypomobility, defined using radiography.

Each study design reflects the specific aims of the research, nevertheless the essential feature of each of the studies was the need to examine how certain tests or examinations could predict a future end-point, e.g. reduction in pain, return to work. The use of the positive or negative likelihood ratio depends on whether the measuring test or instrument needs to rule 'out' a condition, e.g. screening for a behaviour which if not present does not require further investigation, or rule 'in' a condition, e.g. a behaviour is present, therefore the person is at risk (a diagnostic test). Box 5.4 gives some guidance as to how LRs work in practice.

Of note in the studies listed in Table 5.4 is that the majority of the PLRs are not >4 and have wide 95% confidence intervals (CIs), suggesting a limited value for the use of the instruments or measurements, to date.

Construct validity

A construct is an idea or concept, and in the context of measurement properties, construct validity is a process, 'part science and largely art form' (McDowell 2006), which draws the developer and later the reviewer along an evolving set of hypotheses about the new instrument. A series of constructs

---

Box 5.4

Likelihood ratios and clinical practice – how do they work?

The interpretation of reported likelihood ratios for various tests or measurements helps us to decide if the addition of a given test may enhance clinical decision-making.

LRs are used to more accurately establish how performance on an outcome measurement or presence of a series of signs or symptoms will change the probability that a patient will have a condition, e.g. be at risk of falls, improve due to a specific intervention.

Pre-test probability is estimated before the test is used. This may be estimated by using individual clinical judgement based on the history of the patient, or in the case of the studies listed in Table 2.3, the actual prevalence in the study sample.

Thereafter, the likelihood ratio nomogram (Fig. 5.1) may be utilized by:
- Marking the pretest probability on the left of the nomogram
- Marking the LR of the test on the middle line
- Drawing a line through these two points will estimate the post-test probability.

Jaeschke et al (1989) provide the following guide to how to interpret the size of reported LRs, i.e. is the reported LR such that the use of the associated instrument of measurement will better inform practice:
- LRs of >10 or <0.1 may generate large changes in pre and post-test probability
- LRs of 5–10 or 0.1–0.2 generate moderate changes in pre and post-test probability
- LRs of 2–5 and 0.5–0.2 can generate small changes in probability
- LRs of 1–2 and 0.5–1 add rarely important changes to pre-test probability.

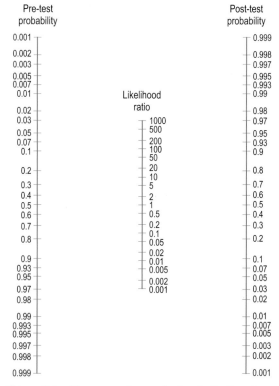

Figure 5.1 • Nomogram for application to likelihood ratios. From Fagan (1975).

are considered, for example in the case of a new instrument to measure functional activities in older people; these might be that:

- The new instrument correlates well with the Barthel Index (convergent validity)
- It measures one or more (in the case of multidimensional instruments) identified domains (factor analysis)
- Older people living in the community who require support services such as home-help and meals-on-wheels would perform less well than those who do not need help from these services or their family/carers in this regard (discriminant, known group validity).

Analysis of the hypotheses around these constructs will either support or otherwise the construct validity of the new instrument. Finch et al (2002) discuss each of the aspects of construct validity mentioned above (convergent validity, etc.) in terms of cross-sectional validity and longitudinal validity. The authors suggest that this taxonomy enables validity associated with a single point in time to be differentiated from that which is associated with change in scores over time. Kirshner and Guyatt (1985) suggest that if instruments are used to evaluate change over time, it is not simply enough to assume that an instrument with cross-sectional validity demonstrates longitudinal validity; this needs to be explicitly examined during the instrument construction. Construct validity, and all it incorporates, differs from the previous types of validity described because it is an ongoing and evolving process, not solved in one or two experimental designs.

Statistical expressions of validity used in construct validity

As outlined above, analysis of face and content validity are primarily discursive and descriptive, more qualitative than quantitative. When statistical analysis of criterion and construct validity is considered, the type of data – nominal, ordinal, interval-ratio – will inform the process.

Factor analysis: content and construct validity

Factor analysis may be applied in the consideration of both content and construct validity. In the former, the items within the instrument, or the

Box 5.5

Factor analysis used in the design of a patient satisfaction scale

Beattie et al (2002) used factor analysis when considering the content validation of a patient satisfaction survey for outpatient physical therapy. Following an initial evaluation, they created an instrument that had 18 questions and two global measures. The questions addressed items such as interaction with the physical therapist, and other matters not related to direct patient care such as location, surroundings, reception, etc.

Using factor analysis, the authors were able to identify that the final instrument would have two components – one relating to the 'patient–therapist' interaction and the other component relating to systems and external aspects. Using this type of analysis, the number of questions was finally reduced from 18 to 10.

sub-scales within a multidimensional inventory are examined to identify how they fit into one or more themes. In the latter, factor analysis may contribute to construct validity by indicating the associations between scales measuring similar constructs and lack of associations with scales measuring different concepts (Streiner & Norman 1989, Reis et al 1991, McDowell 2006). Box 5.5 shows how factor analysis was used in the design of a patient satisfaction scale.

The aim of factor analysis is to simplify a correlation matrix (Kline 1998). In the case of instrument development, this allows the developer to evaluate the themes that emerge from the output of the instrument. For example, Washburn et al (2002) used factor analysis in the development of a scale to measure physical activity for individuals with disabilities. A 12-item scale was administered to 372 subjects with disabilities, and the results on each item were used to compute a 12-item correlation matrix. Factor analysis was utilized to identify if the responses to items within the scale fell into what could be considered 'reasonable and predictable patterns'. The analysis indicated that the scale assessed five dimensions of physical activity and that these items accounted for 63% of the total item variance.

The process of factor analysis is as follows: an inter-item correlation matrix is created, and through principal factor or principle component analysis, the number of variables is reduced to a smaller number of components. This is based on similarities between the items, and is believed to be indicative of the constructs that explain the underlying relationships between the original variables (Roush & Sonstroem 1999). A new correlation matrix is generated, to explore the correlations between the original variables and the new components. This yields a number of outputs (Kline 1998).

- *Factor loadings:* the correlation between the components and the original variables or items. Items with components loadings of >0.3–0.4 and with only one component may be retained (Kline 1998, Washburn et al 2002). Items should 'load on' only one component to be included
- *Eigenvalues* are calculated by squaring and adding the loadings on each factor. Each item has an eigenvalue of 1, hence the factor must have an eigenvalue of >1 if it is to be logically retaining
- *Percentage variance:* the total variance within the correlation matrix that the factor accounts for. It is calculated by dividing the eigenvalue by the number of variables
- *Cumulative percentage variance:* variance accounted for by all the factors. The larger this is, the more variance that is accounted for by the analysis
- *Communality:* squaring and adding the loadings for each item or variable calculates this. It is an indicator of the proportion of variance for each item that each factor accounts for.

Once the initial factor analysis has been computed, there are many different sets of factors which could produce the observed matrix, and factors need to be 'rotated'. Rotation of the factors is a procedure used to clarify the relationships with the correlation matrix, to ensure that the simplest structure is obtained. In terms of identifying which or how many factors should be extracted for rotation, the Scree test is one method that has been proposed (Kline 1998), and is considered the best solution (Kline 1994). The Scree test (Cattell 1966) evaluates a plot of eigenvalues and it is possible to identify from the slope where there is a plateau in the decreasing eigenvalues. One potential flaw in this process is its subjectivity. Figure 5.2 is an example of a Scree test. In this example, six factors would be selected for rotation.

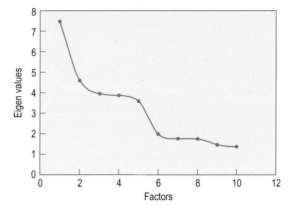

Figure 5.2 • A Scree test.

Can the outcome measure tell the difference between two groups?

Group differences, discriminant validity

When we would like to establish if a new outcome measure will be different in one group of subjects versus another, often two extreme groups are measured and the application of statistical tests for two unrelated groups is reported. These may be unpaired *t*-tests, with confidence intervals, or the Wilcoxon rank sum (two-sample) or Mann–Whitney *U*-tests (Petrie & Sabin 2000); the choice depending on the type of data and the assumption of normal distribution. However, if an instrument is designed to be a diagnostic tool, it is not possible to infer from this type of analysis about finer discriminations (see above).

Summary

Validity is a term widely used when evaluating outcome measures and it can be seen that there are many different forms of validity which give us an insight into the different 'qualifications' of an outcome measure. Table 5.5 summarizes the information in this chapter and may assist when you are making choices and reading about validity.

Table 5.5 Measurement properties and how they inform choice and decision-making – validity

Measurement property	Component of property	Definition	What does it tell us?
Validity	Criterion – concurrent and predictive	Comparing the new outcome measure to a *gold standard*, at one point (concurrent) or at a future point in time (predictive)	How the new measure performs against a more established measure
	Criterion – diagnostic	The accuracy of the outcome measure in identifying whether or not a condition is present	Using scores on the SOM predict a future event, e.g. falls
	Construct, including convergent and discriminant validity	Deeper evaluation of the outcome measure. Developer proposes ideas or constructs about the measure and evaluates the construct	Constructs could be that the SOM measures one or more domains; that it differentiates different groups of patients and others

References

Abbott JH, Mercer SR: Lumbar segmental hypomobility: criterion-related validity of clinical examination items (a pilot study), *New Zealand Journal of Physiotherapy* 31(1):3–9, 2003.

Beattie PF, Pinto MB, Nelson MK, et al: Patient satisfaction with outpatient physical therapy: instrument validation, *Phys Ther* 82(6):557–565, 2002.

Benaim C, Perennou DA, Villy J, et al: Validation of a standardised assessment of postural control in stroke patients, *Stroke* 30:1862–1868, 1999.

Berg KO, Wood-Dauphinee SL, Williams JI, et al: Measuring balance in the elderly: preliminary development of an instrument, *Physiother Can* 41:304–311, 1989.

Bogle Thorbahn LD, Newton RA: Use of the Berg Balance Test to predict falls in elderly persons, *Phys Ther* 76:576–583, 1996.

Bush KW: The statistics of outcome measurement, *Orthopaedic Physical Therapy Clinics of North America* 9(1):55–68, 2000.

Cattell RB: The Scree test for number of factors, *Multivariate Behav Res* 1:140–161, 1966.

Collen FM, Wade DT, Robb GF, et al: The Rivermead Mobility Index: a further development of the Rivermead Motor Assessment, *Int Disabil Stud* 13:50–54, 1991.

Di Fabio RP, Seay R: Use of the 'Fast Evaluation of Mobility, Balance and Fear' in elderly community dwellers: validity and reliability, *Phys Ther* 77 (9):904–917, 1997.

Green BF: A primer of testing, *Am Psychol* 36(10):1001–1011, 1981.

Fagan TJ: Nomogram for Bayes theorem (letter), *N Engl J Med* 293–1257, 1975.

Feinstein A: *Clinometrics*, New Haven, 1987, Yale University Press.

Finch E, Brooks D, Stratford P, et al: *Physical rehabilitation outcome measures – A guide to enhanced clinical decision making*, ed 2, Ontario, 2002, BC Decker.

Fritz JM, Wainner RS, Hicks GE: The use of nonorganic signs and symptoms as a screening tool for return-to-work in patients with acute low back pain, *Spine* 25(15):1925–1931, 2000.

Fritz JM, George SZ: Identifying psychosocial variables in patients with acute work-related low back pain: The importance of fear-avoidance beliefs, *Phys Ther* 82(10):973–984, 2002.

Helmstadter GC: *Principles of psychological measurement*, London, 1966, Metheun & Co Ltd.

Hsieh CL, Hsueh IP, Mao HF: Validity and responsiveness of the Rivermead Mobility Index in stroke patients, *Scand J Rehabil Med* 32:140–142, 2000.

Jaeschke R, Singer J, Guyatt GH: Measurement of health status: ascertaining the minimal clinically important difference, *Control Clin Trials* 10:407–415, 1989.

Kirshner B, Guyatt G: A methodological framework for assessing health indices, *J Chronic Dis* 38(1):27–36, 1985.

Kline P: *An easy guide to factor analysis*, London, 1994, Routledge.

Kline P: *The new psychometrics – science, psychology and measurement*, London, 1998, Routledge.

Kokko SM, Paltamaa J, Ahola E, et al: The assessment of functional ability in patients with Parkinson's disease: The PLM-tests and three clinical tests, *Physiother Res Int* 2:29–45, 1997.

Mao HF, Hseuh IP, Tang PF, et al: Analysis and comparison of the psychometric properties of three balance measures for stroke patients, *Stroke* 33:1022–1027, 2002.

McDowell I: *Measuring Health, A guide to Rating Scales and Questionnaires*, ed 2, New York, 2006, Oxford University Press.

Nilsson LM, Carlsson JY, Brimby G, Nordholm LA: Assessment of walking, balance and sensorimotor performance of hemiparetic patients in the acute stage after stroke, *Physiother Theory Pract* 14:149–157, 1998.

Petrie A, Sabin C: *Medical statistics at a glance*, Oxford, 2000, Blackwell Science.

Piotrowski A, Cole J: Clinical measures of balance and functional assessments in elderly persons, *Aust J Physiother* 40:183–188, 1994.

Platt W, Bell B, Kozak J: Physiotherapy Functional Mobility Profile. A tool for measuring functional outcome in chronic care clients, *Physiother Can* Winter. 47–74, 1998.

Prosser L, Canby A: Further validation of the Elderly Mobility Scale for measurement of mobility of hospitalised elderly, *Clin Rehabil* 11:338–343, 1997.

Reis AL, Kaplan RM, Blumberg E: Use of factor analysis to consolidate multiple outcome measures in chronic obstructive disease, *J Clin Epidemiol* 44(6):497–503, 1991.

Reuben DB, Siu AL: An objective measure of physical function of elderly outpatients. The Physical Performance Test, *J Am Geriatr Soc* 38:1105–1112, 1990.

Riddle D, Stratford PW, Binkley J: Sensitivity to change of the Roland-Morris Back Pain Questionnaire: Part 2, *Phys Ther* 78(11):1197–1207, 1998.

Riddle DL, Stratford PW: Interpreting validity indexes for diagnostic tests: an illustration using the Berg Balance Test, *Phys Ther* 79(10):939–948, 1999.

Roush SE, Sonstroem RJ: Development of the physical therapy outpatient satisfaction survey (PTOPS), *Phys Ther* 79(2):159–170, 1999.

Shumway-Cook A, Baldwin M, Polissar NL, et al: Predicting the probability for falls in community-dwelling older adults, *Phys Ther* 71:812–819, 1997.

Smith R: Validation and reliability of the Elderly Mobility Scale, *Physiotherapy* 80(11):744–747, 1994.

Stevenson TJ, Garland SJ: Standing balance during internally produced perturbations in subjects with hemiplegia: validation of the balance scale, *Arch Phys Med Rehabil* 77:656–661, 1996.

Stratford PW, Binkley J, Riddle D, et al: Sensitivity to change of the Roland-Morris Back Pain Questionnaire: Part 1, *Phys Ther* 78(11):1186–1195, 1998.

Streiner DL, Norman GR: *Health Measurement Scales. A Practical Guide to their Development and Use*, Oxford, 1989, Oxford University Press.

Sutlive TG, Mitchell SD, Maxfield SN, et al: Identification of individuals with patellofemoral pain whose symptoms improved after a combined program of foot orthosis use and modified activity: a preliminary investigation, *Phys Ther* 84(1):49–61, 2004.

Tinetti ME: Performance-oriented assessment of mobility problems in elderly patients, *J Am Geriatr Soc* 34:119–126, 1986.

Usuda S, Araya K, Umehara K, et al: Construct validity of functional balance scale in stroke patients, *Journal of Physical Therapy Science* 10:53–56, 1998.

Washburn RA, Weimo Z, McAuley E, et al: The Physical Activity Scale for individuals with physical disabilities: development and evaluation, *Arch Phys Med Rehabil* 83:193–200, 2002.

Werneke MW, Hart DL: Categorizing patients with occupational low back pain by use of the Quebec Task Force Classification System versus Pain Pattern Classification Procedures: discriminant and predictive validity, *Phys Ther* 84(3):243–255, 2004.

Wolf SL, Catlin PA, Gage K, et al: Establishing the reliability and validity of measurements of walking time using the Emory Functional Ambulation Profile, *Phys Ther* 79:1122–1133, 1999.

Measuring change

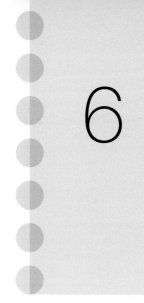

CHAPTER CONTENTS

Introduction

When designing an outcome measurement (OM), the designers may or may not have investigated whether the OM can capture change. The ability of an OM to measure change is often referred to as the *responsiveness* of an OM. How responsive an OM actually is can be measured in a variety of different ways. The methods used may or may not take into consideration whether a patient or client thinks the change is relevant to them.

When choosing an OM for practice, it is important to establish whether responsiveness has been evaluated because this will enable you to decide whether this instrument will actually measure change in your patient/client. If the OM cannot measure change that occurs, it may be difficult to explain that change is taking place and in turn, it may be hard to justify your intervention or service.

Chapter outline

This chapter discusses ways of establishing if an OM can measure change over time and how this property can be reported using descriptive and statistical methods.

The debate about concepts – measuring change – validity or not?

There is unresolved debate in the literature about where the ability of an instrument to measure change falls in the domains of measurement properties. Some authors suggest that the responsiveness or sensitivity to change of an instrument is a separate measurement property and others believe it is part of the art–science continuum of activities that is incorporated in the investigation and evaluation of construct validity (Ch. 5) (Guyatt et al 1987, Hays & Hadorn 1992, Stratford et al 1996). Guyatt et al (1987) support the thesis that measurement responsiveness/sensitivity is a property separate to validity and reliability since it is possible to have a measure that is reliable but not responsive, responsive but not valid and unreliable but yet responsive. Hays and Hadorn (1992) respond to the thesis of Guyatt et al (1987) and suggest that while all of these situations are indeed possible, the artificial distinction between responsiveness/sensitivity may arise from the desire to decide whether measurement instruments are

DOI: 10.1016/B978-0-443-06915-4.00006-1

either valid or not. The authors suggest that validity is in fact an ongoing iterative process and degrees of validity exist. Stratford (1996), in a paper describing the various methods that may be employed to establish measurement sensitivity/responsiveness and the analytical methods that may be employed, opts for including sensitivity/responsiveness as one component of validity. To a certain extent, where sensitivity/responsiveness is placed may be irrelevant as long as the property is examined. Cole et al (1995) note that for many outcome measures used by physiotherapists, a full examination of measurement properties has not been completed and Liang (1995) notes that sensitivity/responsiveness has had the least study. This is changing with increasing numbers of studies reporting on the responsiveness of outcome measured. We have included it in a separate chapter in this book to aid in clarity of describing the various concepts in measurement properties.

The debate about words – measuring change – responsiveness or sensitivity?

There is also ongoing debate on the subject of sensitivity versus responsiveness and which of the two terms to use (Fritz 1999, Stratford 1999, Finch et al 2002). Kirshner and Guyatt first referred to 'responsiveness' as the power of the test to detect clinically relevant change (Kirshner and Guyatt 1985). The two terms have been further defined by Liang (1995) as:

- Sensitivity: the ability to measure any change in a state
- Responsiveness: the ability to measure clinically meaningful or important change.

The author adds that responsiveness implies that the change is noticeable to the patient or health professional and may allow for the person to perform a functional task more efficiently or with less pain or difficulty (Liang 2000). It is the term responsiveness that is widely used in physiotherapy literature (Stratford et al 1996, Wright et al 1998, Hammond 1999, Finch et al 2002) and as such, it will be used throughout this text.

Studying responsiveness

If you were designing a study to consider responsiveness, you could go about it in a number of ways that

have been outlined by Stratford et al (1996) in Figure 6.1.

There are some pros and cons to each design. Design 1 does not take into consideration the situation where there is no change in the patient from T1 to T2. This may be because the patient's condition simply does not change but also may be that change occurs but the measurement is not sensitive enough to capture this change. Second, it does not allow for the review of the measurement's ability in patients who are stable. Design 2 may underestimate the amount of random variability that occurs in patients whose health status is stable; due to the fact that the time spent measuring this may not be sufficiently long enough. Difficulties arise with Design 3 if an established and effective treatment is not available and also with the ethics of not providing such a treatment to a group of patients. In the case of Design 4, it is possible that two groups of patients with a differing temporal component will not actually exist within the group of patients for whom the measurement is designed, e.g. the OM may be designed for patients with acute pain and not for those with chronic pain. The main limitation in Design 5 is identifying another measure, which has a criterion standard for change.

What is interesting about these designs is that in many cases, the view of the patient or client about whether their condition has changed is not considered. However, in Design 5, both the views of the patient or client as well as that of the treating therapist may be applied as the external criterion.

Reporting responsiveness

There are a variety of different ways reported when the responsiveness of a measurement is being analysed (Liang 1995, Taylor et al 2006, Bohannon & Landes 2004, Lee et al 2006). All give an indication of how good the outcome measure is in measuring change. They include:

- Standardized response mean
- Effect size
- Relative efficiency
- Receiver operator characteristic curve.

Standardized response mean and the effect size

The standardized response mean (SRM) is the mean change in scores taken at two time points, divided by the standard deviation of the changes (Liang 1995).

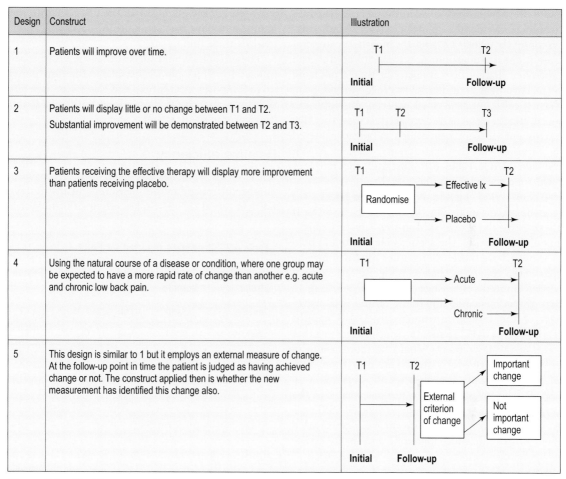

Figure 6.1 • Studying responsiveness. (Adapted from Stratford et al 1996).

The effect size (ES) provides a ratio of the 'signal to noise' within measurement scores on a particular instrument, where the 'signal' is the change that occurs due to intervention and the 'noise' is the level of inherent variability within the outcome measurement. The ES has been used in conjunction with Design 1 in Figure 6.1. Using the standard deviation of baseline scores as a measure of the variance within the data, i.e. noise and the change in scores from admission to discharge as the 'signal', this ratio may be calculated.

Examples of how the effect size has been reported in rehabilitation outcome measures are listed in Box 6.1.

Liang et al (1990) compared the responsiveness of five health status instruments for orthopaedic evaluation: Arthritis Impact Scale (AIMS), Functional Status Index (FSI), Health Assessment Questionnaire (HAQ), Index of Well Being (IWB), and the Sickness Impact Profile (SIP).

A total of 38 participants, 2 weeks prior to hip (55%) or knee (45%) arthroplasty, and at 3, 12 and 15 months after surgery were included in the

Box 6.1

Effect size in rehabilitation outcome measures

Wright et al (1998) measured effect size for both the Rivermead Mobility Index with the Barthel Index and noted effects sizes of 1 and 0.87, respectively. Stokes et al (2003) noted effect sizes of 0.9 for the Elderly Mobility Scale and 0.8 for the Barthel Index.

Effect sizes reported by Bohannon and Landes (2004) for the 3-item and 10-item [20 point] Barthel Index were 2.79 and 3.19, respectively.

study. Responses were divided into 'early' response (baseline: 3 months postoperatively) and 'net' response (baseline: 12 and 15 months postoperatively). The five questionnaires were gathered at each time point. Rather than evaluate the total score from each instrument, four domains were identified: pain, global health (original total scores), mobility and social functioning, and compared across the five instruments, except pain which is only considered by three of the five instruments, namely AIMS, FSI and HAQ. Table 6.1 illustrates the range of SRM reported by the authors.

Cohen's (1977) guide to interpreting effect sizes (see above) was applied by the authors to the SRM. If we evaluate the above SRM in the light of Cohen's guideline (Box 6.1), the sections highlighted in bold in Table 6.1 are those where either the SRM may be considered to be less than a 'moderate' effect, suggesting limited responsiveness. It is interesting to note the influence of timeframe on the responsiveness of the various instruments, i.e. 0–3 months (early) versus 0–12/15 months (net), suggesting that some of the instruments would be more useful in capturing change over a short period of time. This is consistent with the findings of Benaim et al (1999) who investigated the responsiveness of the Postural Assessment Scale for Stroke (PASS) in a group of participants with acute stroke. They divided their sample into mild, moderate and severe stroke

and reported the effect size of the PASS for different numbers of days post-stroke (DAS). Table 6.2 summarizes their findings.

These results would suggest that the PASS is best utilized for all people with stroke in the time period up to 3 months after stroke and thereafter, it is possibly not responsive in those people with mild disability after stroke (Box 6.2).

Relative efficiency

Relative efficiency has also been used to consider a number of rehabilitation measurement instruments (Wright et al 1998, Stokes et al 2003). Wright

Table 6.2 Effect sizes reported for PASS

Days after stroke	Total sample	Mild	Moderate	Severe
14–30	0.89	0.60	1.14	1.01
30–90	0.64	0.29	0.5	1.02
90–180	**0.31**	**0.34**	**0.29**	**0.36**
14–90	1.07	0.76	1.18	1.51
14–180	1.12	0.85	1.20	1.54

Adapted from Benaim et al (1999).

Table 6.1 SRM for five orthopaedic measurement instruments

	Pain	Global health	Mobility	Social
Arthritis Impact Scale (early)	1.11	0.88	1.01	**0.17**
Arthritis Impact Scale (net)	1.15	1.36	1.41	**0.39**
Functional Status Index (early)	1.08	**0.40**	0.78	**0.54**
Functional Status Index (net)	1.00	0.61	0.84	**0.51**
Health Assessment Questionnaire (early)	0.95	**0.33**	0.57	**0.35**
Health Assessment Questionnaire (net)	0.89	1.00	0.84	0.98
Index of Wellbeing (early)	N/A	1.13	0.68	**0.34**
Index of Wellbeing (net)	N/A	0.88	0.91	0.82
Sickness Impact Profile (early)	N/A	0.71	0.94	0.51
Sickness Impact Profile (net)	N/A	1.11	1.10	0.93

Adapted from Liang et al (1990).

Box 6.2

How do we interpret these results for clinical practice?

Cohen (1977) notes that effect sizes that are >0.8 suggest that the measurement instrument is responsive to clinical change. Effect sizes of <0.2 should be interpreted as small and 0.5 as moderate. So, if we are deciding to use an OM in clinical practice and want to be sure it will be responsive to change, the reported effect size will be an important characteristic to consider – the larger the better.

Lee et al (2006) investigated the responsiveness of the Fear-avoidance Beliefs Questionnaire and reported it to be 'moderate' for adults with neck pain – the effect size reported in the paper was 0.32.

---

et al (1998) and Stokes et al (2003) both evaluated the mobility scales and compared them with the Barthel Index, considered a *gold standard* in measurement of functional status. Relative efficiency (Liang et al 1985) is a method of comparing a number of measurement instruments with a view to identifying the relative responsiveness. Depending on the output of the instrument, e.g. whether the data is ordinal or interval a *t* or *z* score is obtained by comparing admission and discharge scores, or indeed scores from any other two designated time points. Relative efficiency is calculated using the following formula:

$$\text{Relative efficient (X versus Y)} = \left({}^{t}X/{}^{t}Y\right)^2$$

A relative efficiency score of 1 would indicate that X is equally as responsive as Y, a score of >1 would suggest that X was more responsive than Y and a score of <1 that Y was more responsive that X. Using this analysis, it has been demonstrated that both the Rivermead Mobility Index and the Elderly Mobility Scale are more responsive than the Barthel Index in older people participating in rehabilitation programmes (Stokes et al 2003, Wright et al 1998). Liang et al (1985) compared the relative efficiency of the AIMS, HAQ, IWB and SIP to the FSI (see above, same sample). The relative efficiencies reported for each of the four domains were as follows:

- Mobility: AIMS (0.85), HAQ (0.48), IWB (0.45), SIP(1.11)
- Pain: AIMS (0.79), HAQ (0.57)
- Social: AIMS (0.18), HAQ (0.62), IWB (0.54), SIP (0.74)

- Global: AIMS (4.12), HAQ (1.15), IWB (7.50), SIP (3.51).

Suggesting that for measuring change in global health, each of the other four instruments is more responsive than the Functional Status Index.

Receiver operator characteristic curves

Receiver operator characteristic (ROC) curves, used in the context of considering the responsiveness of change scores in an instrument or scale between two time points, investigate the sensitivity and specificity (Ch. 5) of the change scores in comparison with an external *gold standard* or criterion of important change (Deyo & Centor 1986).

This means that sensitivity is defined as the number of subjects correctly identified as undergoing important change by a particular scale or instrument and specificity is the number of subjects correctly identified as not having important change. Of note is that 'important change' can be defined by both the patient/client and the therapist. The area under the curve represents the probability of correctly identifying the improved subject from a randomly selected group of improved and unimproved subjects (Stratford et al 1996). A ROC curve can be presented for varying cut-off points.

The area under the curve ranges from 0.5 (no accuracy in detecting improved from unimproved) to 1.0 (perfect accuracy) (Deyo & Centor 1986). Stratford et al (1998) reviewed the responsiveness of the Roland-Morris Questionnaire in 226 subjects who presented with a current episode of low back pain of <6 weeks' duration. The Roland-Morris Questionnaire was measured at baseline and following 3–6 weeks of physiotherapy. Clinician and patient rating of global rating of 'important change' ranged from –7 (deterioration) to +7 (improvement) and a mean clinician and patient global rating score of 5 was considered to represent an important amount of change. This represented the external *gold standard* in Design 5 and 63% of the sample was classified as having changed an important amount. The area under the ROC curve result for the RMQ was 0.84. This suggests that the RMQ had a high level of accuracy in identifying people who had demonstrated 'important change'.

Davidson and Keating (2002) compared the responsiveness of the

- Modified Oswestry Disability Questionnaire (mODC)
- Quebec Back Pain Disability Scale (QBPD)

- Roland-Morris Disability Questionnaire
- Waddell Disability Index
- Physical health scale of the SF-36

in patients undergoing physiotherapy (PT) for low back pain. Measurements were taken at initial consultation and after 6 weeks. External criterion for improvement was if the patient rated their back pain as 'completely gone', 'much better', or 'better' at follow-up. Area under the ROC ranged from 0.73–0.78 for the scales; no significant difference was noted between the ROC curve results for each scale. This is consistent with the results of a similar study comparing the mODC and the QBPD scale in a group ($n = 67$) of subjects with acute, work-related low back pain, also having PT intervention (Fritz & Irrgang 2001). The authors found no difference between the area under the curve (AUC) for the two scales (mODC-0.94, QBPD-0.87). Wagner et al (1993) also employed this method when comparing health status measures in older adults. Self-reported health status measures such as number of restricted activity days, number of days spent in bed due to illness or injury, a physical limitations scale, self-evaluated health and a scale indicating psychological well-being were employed and measured at baseline and 1 year later. The external criterion was an episode of hospitalization or major illness. The results are presented by comparing the area under the ROC curve obtained for each measure to a hypothetical result of 0.5, since this would represent a non-responsive measure. The most responsive health status measures were 'days spent in bed' and 'restricted activity days' and the 'physical activity measure', all of whose area under the ROC curve was significantly different to 0.5.

Summary

The responsiveness of an outcome measure tells us how accurate it may be in capturing change in a patient's status over time. A variety of ways can be used to evaluate responsiveness and a number of statistical methods are also reported. The choice of which analysis to use is dependent on the design of the study and the type of data gathered. In 1995, Liang suggested that to date, no one method has become standard; McDowell (2006) states that there is still no clear consensus.

How can I use this information in my practice?

- Look closely at the OMs you are using and see what research has been done on their responsiveness. Using the information above, you will be able to decide if the outcome measurement is able to measure change in your groups of patients.
- If it is, you might want to also check the minimal detectable change so that you know what change in scores should occur to represent real change (see Ch. 4).
- If no work has been done on the responsiveness of the outcome measurement you may wish to review its use. Could you design a study for your patient/clients? Could you seek funding for such a study, perhaps working with your local research office or university?
- Do you need to change to another outcome measurement? And before you do, investigate its qualifications with respect to responsiveness.

References

Benaim C, Perennou DA, Villy J, et al: Validation of a standardised assessment of postural control in stroke patients, *Stroke* 30: 1862–1868, 1999.

Bohannon R, Landes M: Reliability, validity and responsiveness of a 3-item Barthel for characterizing the physical function of patients hospitalized after acute stroke, *J Neurol Phys Ther* 24(3): 110–113, 2004.

Cohen J: *Statistical power analysis for the behavioural sciences*, New York, 1977, Academic Press.

Cole B, Finch E, Gowland C, Mayo N: In: Basmajian J (ed). *Physical rehabilitation outcome measures*, Toronto, 1995, Health and Welfare Canada and Canadian Physiotherapy Association.

Davidson M, Keating JL: A comparison of five low back pain disability questionnaires: reliability and responsiveness, *Phys Ther* 82(1): 8–24, 2002.

Deyo RA, Centor RM: Assessing the responsiveness of functional scales to clinical change: an analogy to

diagnostic test performance, *J Chronic Dis* 39:897–906, 1986.

Finch E, Brooks D, Stratford P, et al: *Physical rehabilitation outcome measures – A guide to enhanced clinical decision making*, ed 2, Ontario, 2002, BC Decker.

Fritz JM: Sensitivity to change (letter), *Phys Ther* 79(4):420–421, 1999.

Fritz JM, Irrgang JJ: A comparison of a modified Oswestry Low Back Pain Disability Questionnaire and the Quebec Back Pain Disability Scale, *Phys Ther* 81(2):776–788, 2001.

Guyatt G, Walter S, Norman G: Measuring changes over time: the usefulness of evaluative instruments, *J Chronic Dis* 40:171–178, 1987.

Hammond R: Why an outcome measures database? *Physiotherapy* 85(5): 234–235, 1999.

Hays RD, Hadorn D: Responsiveness to change: an aspect of validity, not a separate dimension, *Qual Life Res* 1:73–75, 1992.

Kirshner B, Guyatt G: A methodological framework for assessing health indices, *J Chronic Dis* 38(1):27–36, 1985.

Lee KC, Chiu T, Lam TH: Psychometric properties of the Fear-Avoidance Beliefs Questionnaire in patients with neck pain, *Clin Rehabil* 20:909–920, 2006.

Liang MH: Longitudinal construct validity: establishment of clinical meaning in patient evaluation instruments, *Med Care* 38 (Suppl 11):II-89–90, 2000.

Liang MH, Cullen KE, Schwartz JA: Comparative measurement efficiency and sensitivity of five health status instruments for arthritis research, *Arthritis Rheum* 28:542–547, 1985.

Liang MH, Fossel AH, Larson MG: Comparison of five health status instruments for orthopaedic evaluation, *Med Care* 28:632–642, 1990.

Liang MH: Evaluating measurement responsiveness, *J Rheumatol* 22:1191–1192, 1995.

McDowell I: *Measuring Health. A guide to Rating Scales and Questionnaires*, ed 2, New York, 2006, Oxford University Press.

Stratford P: Who will decide the efficacy of physiotherapeutic interventions? *Physiotherapy Canada Fall* 235–236: 238, 1999.

Stratford PW, Binkley JM, Riddle DL: Health status measures and analytic methods for assessing change scores, *Phys Ther* 76(10): 1109–1123, 1996.

Stratford PW, Binkley J, Riddle D, et al: Sensitivity to change of the Roland-Morris Back Pain Questionnaire: Part 1, *Phys Ther* 78(11):1186–1195, 1998.

Stokes EK, Jennings A, Lyons M, et al: Measuring change in the physiotherapy rehabilitation of older people – Barthel Index and Elderly Mobility Scale. In *Proceedings of the 14th World Confederation for Physical Therapy*, 2003, p 1944.

Taylor S, Frost H, Taylor A, et al: Reliability and responsiveness of the shuttle walking tests in patients with chronic low back pain, *Physiother Res Int* 6(3):170–178, 2006.

Wagner EH, LaCroix AZ, Grothaus LC, Hecht JA: Responsiveness of health status measures to change among older adults, *Jour Am Geriatr Soc* 41:241–248, 1993.

Wright J, Cross J, Lamb S: Physiotherapy outcome measures for rehabilitation of elderly people. Responsiveness to change of the Rivermead Mobility Index and Barthel Index, *Physiotherapy* 84(5):216–221, 1998.

Section 3

Overview

The purpose of Section 3 is to present a method of appraising outcome measures (OM) for use in clinical practice and to present the results of a review of a number of outcome measures. In so doing, it provides a reference source for practitioners about the outcome measures reviewed but also demonstrates how the appraisal method can be used in clinical practice.

The method for appraising outcome measures is based on one described by Greenhalgh et al (1998); this review method combines a descriptive phase and an evaluative phase. The descriptive phase of the review process allows the potential user to consider a 'high-level' view of the OM. In each chapter in Section 3, the first Table reports on this phase; giving a brief description of each instrument, the source, the groups with whom it can be used or the perspective and its user centredness. While

utility of an instrument is a subjective evaluation, an attempt to describe this is made, including details on equipment and timings. Where it has been possible to obtain permission for authors or copyright holders, the instruments have been reproduced with an acknowledgement in the Appendix. Notwithstanding such permission, the primary sources of each instrument are also provided.

Once this descriptive phase has been completed, and if it seems that the OM is available, appropriate and, in some cases, affordable, the reader is advised to read the second Table in the chapters in Section 3. Section 2 of this book outlines in detail how measurement properties can be analysed and what the results of such analyses can inform in our clinical decision-making. This should be referred to when reading the evaluative phase, i.e. Tables 2 in the various chapters in Section 3.

Measuring mobility

7

CHAPTER CONTENTS

Introduction

For the purposes of this chapter, mobility is defined as the ability to move around an individual's environment. It takes environment in its broadest context; for those with limited mobility, individual environment may simply mean movement in bed and transfers in and out of bed. For those with higher levels of mobility, it includes running and jumping and the Life Space Assessment moves the location beyond the home and into the neighbourhood. The measures of mobility included in this chapter may be linked with the following ICF (WHO 2001) categories:

- d410 Changing basic body position
- d415 Maintaining a body position
- d420 Transferring oneself
- d450 Walking
- d455 Moving around
- d460 Moving around in different locations.

As described in Chapter 3, the checklist reported by Greenhalgh et al (1998) is the basis for the information provided in the tables that accompany this chapter on each outcome measure. Where relationships between variables are described in the context of validity and reliability, the statistical tests employed are co-efficients such as Pearson Product Moment and Spearman's Rank correlation co-efficient unless otherwise stated. Where details of the exact intra-class correlation (ICC) were provided in the primary source, it is included in the table and if not, the abbreviation ICC is used.

© 2011, Elsevier Ltd.
DOI: 10.1016/B978-0-443-06915-4.00007-3

Table 7.1 Emory Functional Ambulation Category (E-FAP) and Modified Emory Functional Ambulation Category (mE-FAP)

Description	Perspective	Language	Availability & publications	User-centredness	Requirements & utility
Initial version – 5 sub-tasks which are timed with a loading for various assistive devices. Modified E-FAP includes both assistive device use and need for manual assistance	Stroke. Measures observed performance in people with stroke – time to walk in 5 different environments	English	Available in Baer & Wolf (2001). See Appendix 1. Wolf et al (1999). Liaw et al (2006)	Observed performance of people with stroke, no user involvement in development. The developers suggest that its use will be helpful to those making decisions about home environment and employment opportunities	Requires hard-surfaced floor, carpet, obstacle course and stairs. Combines a series of relevant components in one instrument

Face/content	Validity		Reliability	Measuring change
	Criteria including concurrent, predictive and diagnostic	Construct including convergent and discriminant	Relative	
Conceptualization described by developers. Further developed to include manual assistance.	E-FAP Concurrent: Compared with Functional Reach (FR) (0.71), Berg Balance Scale (BBS) (−0.6), timed 10 m walk (−0.3). mE-FAP Concurrent: Compared with initial, final and change in BBS (−0.74, −0.70, −0.54) and initial, final and change in Functional Independence Measure (FIM) (−0.66, −0.78, −0.15) mE-FAP Predictive: Admission mE-FAP compared with discharge BI (−0.51) and RMI (−0.78)	E-FAP: Captured difference between people with stroke and age and gender-matched group. mE-FAP: Two studies in people with stroke. E-FAP Convergent: Compared with Barthel Index (BI) (0.76) E-FAP Discriminant: correlation with change scores on IADL (0.30), Spitzer Quality of Life (0.39) and Mini Mental State Examination (MMSE) (0.15) mE-FAP Convergent: Compared with 10 m timed test (admission 0.88, discharge 0.93) and Rivermead Mobility Index (RMI) (admission −0.67, discharge −0.81)	E-FAP: Inter-rater ($n = 28$): ICC (2,1) = 0.98-1.0 mE-FAP: Inter-rater ($n = 7$): ICC = 0.99 Test-re-test ($n = 5$): ICC = 0.99 Inter-rater ($n = 20$): ICC (3,1) ≥0.97	mE-FAP Standardized response mean 1.1

Table 7.2 Hierarchic assessment of balance and mobility (HABAM)

Description	Perspective	Language	Availability & publications	User-centredness	Requirements & utility
3 sections: balance, transfers, mobility. Rasch analysis informs the scoring system	Older adults Measures observed performance in older people – both in- and outpatients	English	Available in Rockwood et al (2008) See Appendix 1 MacKnight & Rockwood (1995, 2000)	Observed performance in older people. The developers suggest that quick, simple instruments that are acceptable to patients are desirable. Provides visual display of performance and score	No specific requirements – provides visual measure of performance in addition to score

Validity		Reliability		Measuring change	
Face/content		Relative			
Scale developed to be hierarchic and performance based by developers, to track progression and recovery in frail older adults. Face validity assessed by Professor of Geriatric Medicine		Inter-rater ($n = 28$): ICC –0.94 Inter-rater ($n = 167$): ICC –0.89–0.91 Test–re-test ($n = 63$): ICC –0.85–0.92		Relative efficiency compared with BI 3.13; Effect size 0.59	

Table 7.3 Elderly Mobility Scale (EMS) and Swedish Modified EMS (Swe mEMS)

Description	Perspective	Language	Availability & publications	User-centredness	Requirements & utility
7-item scale that evaluates mobility and transfers in older people	Older adults, stroke. Measures observed performance	English, Swedish, Dutch	EMS available in Smith (1994), Prosser & Canby (1997), Spilg et al (2001) Swe mEMS available in Linder et al (2006) See Appendix 1 Smith (1994) Cuijpers et al (2004) Nolan et al (2008)	Evaluates performance in older people covering basic requirements for more complex activities of daily living (ADL)	Simple, easy to use in clinical department. Observed performance is scored.

Face/content	Validity	Reliability	Measuring change
	Criteria including concurrent, predictive and diagnostic	Relative	
Initial development was following discussions with physiotherapists working with older people and a review of the literature. Swedish version has been evaluated in people with stroke and modified slightly	English version Concurrent: Comparison with BI (0.962, 0.787) and FIM (0.948) Discriminant: Inpatient group compared with healthy community dwelling sample ($n = 20$, all scored maximum score) Swedish version Concurrent: Comparison with Berg Balance Scale (0.86–0.94) and Motor Assessment Scale Upper Arm Section (0.69–0.88)	Video-recording analysis on nine subjects. Latent class analysis demonstrated good inter-rater ($n = 18$) and intra-rater ($n = 15$). Dutch version: Inter-rater ICC = 0.95–0.97 Intra-rater ICC = 0.97 Bland & Altman limits of agreement 3 points. Swedish version ($n = 30$): Inter-rater ICC 0.98–0.99	Compared with BI and Functional Ambulation Category (FAC) ($n = 395$) – EMS detected a change in scores with a significant difference between admission and discharge score and was more informative than FAC or BI

Table 7.4 Rivermead Mobility Index (RMI) and Modified Rivermead Mobility Index (mRMI)

Description	Perspective	Language	Availability & publications	User-centredness	Requirements & utility
Rivermead Mobility Index (RMI) is a self-reported measure of mobility including 15 items with a score of Yes or No. One of the items is observed. A modified version (mRMI) for physiotherapists is 8-items and a 0–5 scoring system	Stroke, intellectual disability, older adults, adults with neurological disability	English, Italian, German, Dutch	RMI English (2-level) available in Collen et al (1991), Forlander & Bohannon (1999), Ryall et al (2003). mRMI available in Lennon & Johnson (2000). RMI German available in Schindl et al (2000). RMI Italian available in Franchignoni et al (2003). See Appendix 1 Wright et al (1998) Hsieh et al (2000) Rossier & Wade (2001) Green et al (2001) Hsueh et al (2003) Sackley et al (2005) Chen et al (2007) Roorda et al (2008)	Asks the patient/client to report on his/her performance. The tasks included range from limited mobility in bed to running	The patient/client reports on 14 items, and one item – standing unsupported – is observed. If the patient cannot provide the answers, the primary caregiver can report

Continued

Table 7.4 Rivermead Mobility Index (RMI) and Modified Rivermead Mobility Index (mRMI)—cont'd

Validity			Reliability			Measuring Change
Face/content	Criteria including concurrent, predictive and diagnostic	Construct including convergent and discriminant	Relative	Absolute	Internal consistency	
The initial development was iterative. It was informed by a perceived gap in the availability of measures with a suitable range. The first iteration was developed, evaluated on people post-stroke, and this led to a second iteration. The development of the mRMI in stroke employed a consensus exercise of 42 physiotherapists identifying which items they thought were 'essential'. They also commented on the extended scoring system. Thereafter, the mRMI was tested on 30 subjects with stroke. It is scored by direct observation	RMI in chronic stroke: Predictive: Comparison of admission RMI scores to BI at discharge (0.77) RMI and mRMI in stroke: Concurrent: scores on mMRI more closely associated with other performance measure than with RMI Predictive: Relationship between scores on both and BI (0.53–0.83) at 180 days after stroke	RMI in neurological disease: RMI scores statistically different between two groups with different mobility status RMI stroke: The coefficient of scalability is acceptable (>0.6). 'Highly' associated compared with BBS and BI for convergent validity. RMI and mRMI in stroke: Convergent: Relationship between scores on both and BI (0.72–0.89) and at 180 days after stroke	RMI in stroke: Inter-rater ($n = 40$) ICC = 0.92 mRMI in stroke: Inter-rater ($n = 40$) ICC = 0.95	RMI in chronic stroke: Minimal detectable change (MDC_{95}) = 2.2	mRMI: Cronbach's alpha = 0.93	RMI in rehabilitation Effect size 1 Relative efficiency 1.25, better than BI mRMI: Effect size 1.15 RMI and mRMI in stroke: Standardized response mean between 14–30 days −1.14 and 1.31

Table 7.5 High-level Mobility Assessment Tool (HiMAT)

Description	Perspective	Language	Availability & publications	User-centredness	Requirements & utility
This scale was developed because of a lack of scales capturing high levels of mobility. The proposed users for whom it was developed are young people with traumatic brain injury (TBI)	Younger people with TBI	English	Available online See Appendix 1 Williams et al (2004, 2005, 2006)	It is designed for young people with TBI who aim to return to their previous sporting, vocational and civic roles	This scale takes about 5–10 min and observes performance while timing the tasks. There is a minimal mobility requirement of being able to walk for 20 m without an assistive device but orthoses may be worn

Validity	Reliability		
Face/content	Relative	Absolute	Internal consistency
Item generation selection resulted from an iterative design process involving experts in physiotherapy and physical education. Initially 157 items were generated. A 15-item version was further analysed – Rasch analysis and factor analysis. The final scale has 13 items	Test–re-test (n = 20): ICC (2,1) = 0.99 Inter-rater (n = 17): ICC (2,1) = 0.99	MDC_{95} = −2 to +4 (i.e. deterioration in 2 points or improvement in 4 points)	Cronbach's alpha (n = 103) = 0.97

Table 7.6 Physiotherapy Functional Mobility Profile (PFMP) and Physiotherapy Functional Mobility Profile Questionnaire (PFMP-Q)

Description	Perspective	Language	Availability & publications	User-centredness	Requirements & utility
The scale contains 9 items relating to functional mobility, each scored by observation from 1–7. The PFMP-Q is a questionnaire version	Older adults, acute inpatients	English, French	Available in Platt et al (1998), Brosseau et al (1999), Laferrière et al (2001)	The scale was developed for use with older adults who require ongoing 'chronic' care. It can also be used in acute inpatients with a lower functional status	Simple, easy to use. Requires 50 m stretch for walk and 12–14 steps on stairs

	Validity		Reliability	
Face/content	Criteria including concurrent, predictive and diagnostic	Construct including convergent and discriminant	Relative	Internal consistency
Face and content validity were considered during the development phase by using a Delphi technique to achieve professional consensus among a panel of 7 experienced physiotherapists	Older adults: Principal component factor analysis was completed revealing only one dimension, i.e. functional mobility. Acute inpatients: Principal component factor analysis was completed revealing only one dimension, i.e. disability. Convergent: A variable relationship was noted between scores on items as reported by patients and family. Sensitivity and specificity: 0.91 and 0.92 at patient reported questionnaire predicting independence or dependence as observed by physiotherapist. Concurrent: Strong relationship between patient-reported and directly observed status	Older adults: Discriminant: Admission scores were evaluated to ascertain if the PFMP could differentiate between groups of adults admitted from living in the community and those living in institutional care: the scores were significantly different. PFMP scores on discharge were similarly able to also discriminate between different discharge destinations	PFMP: Older adults: Inter-rater reliability evaluated on video-taped recordings of 9 subjects by 7 physiotherapists, ICC = 0.47–0.93. Intra-rater reliability: no significant changes in the scores of the raters. Acute inpatients: Inter-rater ($n = 10$ video-taped subjects) ICC (2,1) = 0.97. Intra-rater ($n = 55$ video-taped subjects) ICC (1,1) = 0.99. PFMP-Q: Intra-rater for patient interview and family ICC (1,1) = 0.95–0.96. Inter-rater for patient interview and family interview ICC (1,1) = 0.83–0.97	Older adults: Cronbach's alpha ($n = 1,127$) = 0.96. Acute inpatients ($n = 55$) = 0.99

Table 7.7 University of Alabama at Birmingham Study of Aging Life Space Assessment (UAB – LSA)

Description	Perspective	Language	Availability & publications	User-centredness	Requirements & utility
The UAB-LSA measures mobility, based on the distance a person has moved through in the previous 4 weeks. LSA can consider the environment – level 1–5; the assistance required and the frequency. LSA-C is a composite of 3 components level $\times$ frequency $\times$ independence	Older adults	English, French French Canadian version of LSA = LSA-F	Available in Peel et al (2005) See Appendix 1 Baker et al (2003) Auger et al (2009)	The scale has various forms; the composite form is reported in this chapter. Various forms can be used for different evaluative purposes including longitudinal studies of ageing	The LSA requires the patient/client to recall the life space used in the previous 4 weeks to diminish the effects of transient illness or other factors that might have a short-term impact on mobility. Peel et al (2005) suggest that declines in life space should be investigated to ascertain if the changes are amenable to intervention. It can be used in interview or by telephone

	Validity			Reliability	
Face/content			Construct including convergent and discriminant	Relative	
Content validity of the French version was completed with the involvement of translators, clinicians and users of power mobility devices			UAB-LSA: Convergent ($n = 306$): correlation with a Short Physical Performance Battery (SPPB) (0.603) and in a larger study ($n = 998$), ADL and IADL and SPPB accounted for 45.5% of the variance in LSA scores	UAB-LSA: Test-re-test – baseline and 2 weeks ($n = 306$): ICC = 0.96 LSA-F: Test-re-test 2-week interval ($n = 40$): ICC = 0.87	

Table 7.8 Trinity Test of Functional Mobility (TTFM)

Description	Perspective	Language	Availability & publications	User-centredness	Requirements & utility
Trinity Test comprises 7 items as follows: Bed rise (0–6); sit to stand (0–6); standing ability and stability (0–13); reach and lift (0–6); bend and reach (0–6); repeated sit to stand (0–8); and gait ability (0–12)	Older adults	English	Available in Stokes & O'Neill (2007) See Appendix 1 Stokes & O'Neill (2010)	The scale was developed for use with older people having rehabilitation	The performance of the older person is observed. It requires basic equipment readily available in a rehabilitation gym. The scores range from very dependent to timed test at the higher end of the scale.

Validity			Reliability			Measuring change
Face/content	Criterion including concurrent, predictive and diagnostic	Construct including convergent and discriminant	Relative	Absolute	Internal consistency	
An iterative design involving expert physiotherapists and a review of the literature yielded the first iteration of the scale which had further evaluation	Principal component factor analysis in a sample of 73 older adults yielded one factor accounting for 70% of the variance: functional mobility	Concurrent: Admission scores on TTFM correlated with admission EMS (0.80), Performance Oriented Assessment Mobility (POAM-Tinetti) (0.86 balance) Predictive: Admission scores on TTFM correlated with discharge EMS (0.65), Performance Oriented Assessment Mobility (POAM-Tinetti) (0.69 balance)	Inter-rater reliability ($n = 15$) % agreement: 97–98.4% (wKappa 0.69–1) Test-re-test ($n = 15$) 93% (wKappa 0.93)	$MDC_{95} = 5.5$	Cronbach's alpha = 0.783	Effect size = 0.64 Relative efficiency compared with EMS (1.75) and POAM-Tinetti (1.50)

Table 7.9 The Activities-specific Balance Confidence Scale (ABC)

Description	Perspective	Language	Availability & publications	User-centredness	Requirements & utility
ABC is a 16-item scale that is scored from 0–100. Responders are asked to consider the 16 items and respond to the question 'how confident are you in doing . . . without losing your balance or becoming unsteady?' The 16 items range from reaching at eye level to walking on an icy road, and include varying levels of possible hazard	Stroke, Multiple Sclerosis (MS), lower limb amputee, older people living in the community or in institutional care	English, French Canadian, Hebrew, Chinese	See Appendix 1 Powell & Myers (1995) Miller et al (2003) Lajoie & Gallagher (2004) Holbein-Jenny et al (2005) Botner et al (2005) Salbach et al (2006) Cattaneo et al (2006) Hsu & Miller (2006) Mak et al (2007) Elboim-Gabizon et al (2008) Talley et al (2008)	The views of older adults were sought in the development of the list of items included. It is a self-reported measure, based on the 0–100% response continuum recommended by Bandura for evaluating self-efficacy	It is simple and easy to use. It takes approx. 10–20 min to complete

Validity			Reliability		Measuring change
Face/content	Criterion including concurrent, predictive and diagnostic	Construct including convergent and discriminant	Relative	Internal consistency	
Both clinicians and older people were asked to name the 10 most important activities essential to independent living 'that while requiring some position change or walking would not normally be hazardous	ABC scores are moderately correlated with: Physical self-efficacy scores (0.49), Fall Efficacy Scale (FES) (−0.33), Timed Up & Go (TUG) (−0.39) in community dwelling older adults. In both	Discriminant: A cut-off score of 67% yielded a sensitivity of 84% and specificity of 87% for correctly classifying fallers in a sample of older people living in the community. In lower limb amputees, scores on the ABC were	Test–re-test ICCs ranging from 0.70 (home care residents) to 0.91 (lower limb amputees)	Cronbach's alpha: In the initial development in a group of older people $(n = 60) = 0.96$ In 50 lower limb amputees = 0.91. In a sample of people with stroke $(n = 77) = 0.94$	In older women living in the community, standardized response mean = 0.05

Continued

Table 7.9 The Activities-specific Balance Confidence Scale (ABC)—cont'd

Validity			Reliability	Measuring change
Face/content	Criterion including concurrent, predictive and diagnostic	Construct including convergent and discriminant	Relative	Internal consistency
to most elderly persons'. Factor analysis of a sample of people with stroke yielded two factors accounting for 68.6% of variance	community dwelling and those living in residences, correlations with Berg Balance Scale (BBS) are 0.57 and 0.55, respectively. In lower limb amputees, ABC scores correlate strongly with a 6 min walk test (−0.72) and TUG (−0.70). Correlations between ABC scores and TUG in MS (−0.38) and gait speed in stroke (−0.36). Correlations between ABC and BBS were 0.48 and 0.36, respectively	significantly lower and could differentiate between groups of mobility device used, cause of amputee and automatic stepping ability. In a sample of users with MS, the scores on ABC were better than those on the Berg Balance Scale, Timed Up & Go or Dynamic Gait Index in differentiating between fallers and non-fallers		

References

Auger C, Demers L, Gélinas I, et al: Developments of a French-Canadian version of the life-space assessment (LSA-F): content validity, reliability and applicability for power mobility device users, *Disability and Rehabilitation: Assistive Technology* 4 (1):31–41, 2009.

Baer HR, Wolf SL: Modified Emory functional ambulation profile: an outcome measure for the rehabilitation of poststroke gait dysfunction, *Stroke* 32:973–979, 2001.

Baker PS, Bodner EV, Allman RM: Measuring life-space mobility in community-dwelling older adults, *J Am Geriatr Soc* 51:1610–1614, 2003.

Botner EM, Miller WC, Eng JJ: Measurement properties of the Activities-specific Balance Confidence Scale among individuals with stroke, *Disabil Rehabil* 27 (4):156–163, 2005.

Brosseau L, Laferrière L, Couroux N, et al: Intra- and inter-rater reliability and factorial validity studies of the Physiotherapy Functional Mobility Profile (PFMP) in acute care patients, *Physiother Theory Pract* 15:147–154, 1999.

Cattaneo D, Regola A, Meotti M: Validity of six balance disorders scales in persons with multiple sclerosis, *Disabil Rehabil* 28(12):789–795, 2006.

Chen HM, Hsieh CL, Lo SK, et al: The test–re-test reliability of 2 mobility performance tests in patients with chronic stroke, *Neurorehabil Neural Repair* 21:347–352, 2007.

Collen FM, Wade DT, Robb GF, et al: The Rivermead Mobility Index: a further development of the Rivermead Motor Assessment, *Int Disabil Stud* 13(2):50–54, 1991.

Cuijpers CJT, Nelissen LH, Lenssen AF: Intra- and inter-rater reliability of the Dutch version of the Elderly Mobility Scale in the frail elderly, *Nederlands Tijdschrift Voor Fysiotherapie* 114 (4):110–113, 2004.

Elboim-Gabizon M, Barzilai N, Chemel I, et al: Validity and reliability of the Hebrew version of the Activities-specific Balance Confidence Scale, *Journal of the Israeli Physical Therapy Society (JIPTS)* 10(2):32, 2008.

Forlander DA, Bohannon RW: Rivermead Mobility Index: a brief review of research to date, *Clin Rehabil* 13:97–100, 1999.

Franchignoni F, Tesio L, Benevolo E, et al: Psychometric properties of the Rivermead Mobility Index in Italian stroke rehabilitation inpatients, *Clin Rehabil* 17:273–282, 2003.

Green J, Forster A, Young J: A test–re-test reliability study of the Barthel Index, the Rivermead Mobility Index, the Nottingham extended Activities of Daily Living Scale and Frenchay Activities Index in stroke patients, *Disabil Rehabil* 23(15):670–676, 2001.

Greenhalgh J, Long AF, Brettle AJ, et al: Reviewing and selecting outcome measures for use in routine practice, *J Eval Clin Pract* 4(4):339–350, 1998.

Holbein-Jenny MA, Billek-Sawhney B, Beckman E, et al: Balance in personal care home residents: A comparison of the Berg Balance Scale, the Multi-Directional Reach Test, and the Activities-Specific Balance Confidence Scale, *J Geriatr Phys Ther* 28(2):48, 2005.

Hsueh IP, Wang CH, Sheu CF, et al: Comparison of psychometric properties of three mobility measures for patients with stroke, *Stroke* 34:1741–1745, 2003.

Hsieh CL, Hsueh IP, Mao HF: Validity and responsiveness of the Rivermead Mobility Index in Stroke patients, *Scand J Rehabil Med* 32:140–142, 2000.

Hsu PC, Miller WC: Reliability of the Chinese version of the Activities-specific Balance Confidence Scale, *Disabil Rehabil* 28(20):1287–1292, 2006.

Laferrière L, Brosseau L, Narezny M, et al: Reliability and the validity of the physiotherapy functional mobility profile questionnaire, *Physiother Theory Pract* 17:217–228, 2001.

Lajoie Y, Gallagher SP: Predicting falls within the elderly community: comparison of postural sway, reaction time, the Berg balance scale and the Activities-specific Balance Confidence (ABC) Scale for comparing fallers and non-fallers, *Arch Gerontol Geriatr* 38:11–26, 2004.

Lennon S, Johnson L: *The modified Rivermead Mobility Index: validity & reliability*, 22(18):833–839, 2000.

Liaw LJ, Hsieh CL, Lo SK, et al: Psychometric properties of the modified Emory functional ambulation profile in stroke patients, *Clin Rehabil* 20(5):429–437, 2006.

Linder A, Winkvist L, Nilsson L, et al: Evaluation of the Swedish version of the Modified Elderly Mobility Scale (Swe M-EMS) in patients with acute stroke, *Clin Rehabil* 20:584–597, 2006.

MacKnight C, Rockwood K: Rasch analysis of the hierarchical assessment of balance and mobility (HABAM), *J Clin Epidemiol* 53:1242–1247, 2000.

MacKnight C, Rockwood K: A hierarchical assessment of balance and mobility, *Age Ageing* 24:126–130, 1995.

Mak MK, Lau AL, Law FS, et al: Validation of the Chinese translated Activities-specific Balance Confidence Scale, *Arch Phys Med Rehabil* 88:496–503, 2007.

Miller WC, Deathe AB, Speechley M: Psychometric properties of the Activities-Specific Balance Confidence Scale among individuals with a lower-limb amputation, *Arch Phys Med Rehabil* 87:656–661, 2003.

Nolan JS, Remilton LE, Green MM: The Reliability and Validity of the Elderly Mobility Scale in the acute hospital setting, *Internet Journal of Allied Health Sciences and Practice* 6(4): 2008.

Platt W, Bell B, Kozak J: Physiotherapy Functional mobility profile: a tool for measuring functional outcome in chronic care clients, *Physiother Can* 47:74, 1998.

Peel C, Sawyer- Baker P, Roth DL, et al: Assessing Mobility in Older Adults: The U A B Study of Aging Life-Space Assessment, *Phys Ther* 85:1008–1019, 2005.

Powell LE, Myers AM: The Activities-specific Balance Confidence Scale (ABC) Scale, *J Gerontol* 50A(1): M28–M34, 1995.

Prosser L, Canby A: Further validation of the Elderly Mobility Scale for measurement of mobility of hospitalized elderly people, *Clin Rehabil* 11:338–343, 1997.

Rockwood K, Rockwood MRH, Andrew MK, et al: Reliability of the hierarchical assessment of balance and mobility in frail older adults, *J Am Geriatr Soc* 56:1213–1217, 2008.

Roorda LD, Green J, De Kluis KR, et al: Excellent cross-cultural validity, intra-test reliability and construct validity of the Dutch Rivermead Mobility Index in patients after stroke undergoing rehabilitation, *J Rehabil Med* 40(9):727–732, 2008.

Rossier P, Wade DT: Validity and reliability comparison of 4 mobility measures in patients presenting with neurologic impairment, *Arch Phys Med Rehabil* 82:9–13, 2001.

Ryall NH, Eyres SB, Neumann VC, et al: Is the Rivermead Mobility Index appropriate to measure mobility in lower limb amputees, *Disabil Rehabil* 25(3):143–153, 2003.

Sackley C, Richardson P, McDonnell K, et al: The reliability of balance, mobility and self-care measures in a population of adults with a learning disability known to a physiotherapy service, *Clin Rehabil* 19:216–223, 2005.

Salbach NM, Mayo NE, Hanley JA, et al: Psychometric evaluation of the original and Canadian French version of the Activities-specific Balance Confidence Scale among people with stroke, *Arch Phys Med Rehabil* 87:1597–1604, 2006.

Schindl MR, Forstner C, Kern H, et al: Evaluation of a German version of the Rivermead Mobility Index (RMI) in acute and chronic stroke patients, *Eur J Neurol* 7:523–528, 2000.

Smith R: Validation and reliability of the Elderly Mobility Scale, *Physiotherapy* 80(11):744–747, 1994.

Spilg EG, Martin BJ, Mitchell SL: A comparison of mobility assessments in a geriatric day hospital, *Clin Rehabil* 15:296–300, 2001.

Stokes EK, O'Neill D: Towards the development of an outcome measure for functional mobility of older people – an evaluation of face and content validity of the Trinity Test, *Physiotherapy Ireland* 28(2):58–69, 2007.

Stokes EK, O'Neill: Trinity Test of Functional Mobility: preliminary report of measurement properties (in preparation), 2010.

Talley KMC, Wyman JF, Gross CR: Psychometric properties of the Activities-specific Balance Confidence Scale and the Survey of activities and fear of falling in older women, *J Am Geriatr Soc* 56:328–333, 2008.

Williams GP, Greenwood KM, Robertson VJ, et al: High-Level Mobility Assessment Tool (HiMat): interrater reliability, re-test reliability, and internal consistency, *Phys Ther* 86(3):395–400, 2006.

Williams GP, Robertson V, Greenwood KM, et al: The high-level mobility assessment tool (HiMat) for traumatic brain injury Part 1: Item generation, *Brain Inj* 19 (11):925–932, 2005.

Williams GP, Robertson V, Greenwood KM, et al: The high-level mobility assessment tool (HiMAT) for traumatic brain injury Part 2: Content validity and discriminability, *Brain Inj* 19(10):833–843, 2004.

Wolf SL, Catlin PA, Gage K, et al: Establishing the reliability and validity of measurements of walking time using the Emory functional ambulation profile, *Phys Ther* 79 (12):1122–1133, 1999.

WHO: *International Classification of Functioning, Disability and Health*, Geneva, 2001, World Health.

Wright J, Cross J, Lamb S: Physiotherapy outcome measures for rehabilitation of elderly people, *Physiotherapy* 84 (5):216–221, 1998.

Measuring physical activity

CHAPTER CONTENTS

Introduction

With the possible exception of diet, we know of no single intervention with greater promise than physical activity to reduce the risk of virtually all chronic diseases simultaneously (Booth et al 1997).

Regular, health-enhancing physical activity can have life-long health benefits and the public health message is that physical activity levels should be higher. Barriers to taking physical activity may change as we age (SLAN & HBSC 2006) but nonetheless, the benefits exist throughout the lifespan. There are three main forms of physical activity: competitive sport (for fun or personal gain including a sense of fulfilment); structured exercise (which tends to be setting dependent); and active living (e.g. walking or cycling to the shops) (Woods 2009).

Physical activity can be measured in two ways, through self-reported questionnaires or diaries and directly by accelerometers. Accelerometers 'measure bodily movement or acceleration by evaluating movement in one (uniaxial) to three (triaxial) directions'. The axes of movement are vertical in a uniaxial accelerometer; horizontal and sagittal are collected in a triaxial accelerometer. Accelerations are converted into a raw data output of activity count values and steps. Measurement intervals can range from 5 s to 1 min depending on the device used. Combining the output of some accelerometers with data on gender, height, weight and age can yield energy expenditure data such as metabolic equivalent units (METs). The number of steps accumulated per unit of time is used to estimate intensity level and can be classified as light-, moderate- and vigorous-intensity activity using reported cut-off points. Cut-off points may be affected by anthropometric measurements so they may need to be population specific (Rowlands et al 2004).

Some of the challenges of accelerometers in clinical practice are as follows:

* Not all accelerometers are valid for use with older people or for people with neurological disability who may have altered gait patterns.
* Accelerometers may under-estimate energy expenditure, especially when workload increases (Resnick et al 2001) and those worn at the waist or on the lower limb will not measure upper limb activities.
* Using the output of uniaxial accelerometers in children may under-estimate the level of activity because, while most activity in adults will be captured in the vertical plane, some activities of children may not occur in this plane and data from the horizontal and sagittal planes will capture such activities.

DOI: 10.1016/B978-0-443-06915-4.00008-5

Survey instruments or exercise logs also have limitations such as relying on recall, over or under-estimation of activity levels. Outlined below are details on two commonly used, commercially available accelerometers and three survey instruments for evaluating physical activity levels in various groups of patients/clients.

As described in Chapter 3, the checklist reported by Greenhalgh et al (1998) is the basis for the information provided in the tables that accompany this chapter on each outcome measure. Where relationships between variables are described in the context of validity and reliability, the statistical tests employed are co-efficients such as Pearson Product Moment and Spearman's Rank correlation co-efficient unless otherwise stated. Where details of the exact intra-class correlation (ICC) were provided in the primary source, it is included in the table and if not, the abbreviation ICC is used.

Table 8.1 StepWatch™ Monitor – Step Activity Monitor (SAM)

Description	User groups	Availability & publications	User-centredness utility
The StepWatch™ Monitor was proposed by Dr D G Smith in 1991. It is a small device worn over the lateral malleolus. It detects and counts steps. The sensor developed for SAM is an accelerometer and an electronic filter. The sensitivity of the sensor for step counting can be adjusted by varying two filtering parameters – cadence and motion. It is suitable for use in populations with mobility disorders and slower walking speeds.	Healthy adults Obese adults Stroke Parkinson's disease Older adults living in the community and in assisted living environments Adults following lower limb surgery Incomplete spinal cord injury Duchenne muscular dystrophy Able-bodied children and adolescents	www.orthocareinnovations.com Coleman et al (1999) Shepherd et al (1999) Resnick et al (2001) Macko et al (2002) Haeuber et al (2004) McDonald et al (2005a, 2005b) Bergman et al (2007) Bowden & Behrman (2007) Mudge & Stott (2007, 2008) Storti et al (2008) Busse et al (2009)	The StepWatch™ Monitor is worn slightly above the ankle and is attached using a Velcro strap. It is used in conjunction with a PC, software and a docking station. Prior to providing the SAM to a user, it is programmed to take account of the individual's height, walking speed and ankle motion. The recorded data is downloaded to a PC and the software provides graphical and text analyses of the data.

Validity			Reliability	
Face/content	Criteria validity accuracy	Construct	Relative	

Face/content	Criteria validity accuracy	Construct	Relative
The SAM measures step counts and an initial paper reports that its development was to 'overcome the limitations of the previously available long-term activity monitors'. Step count is considered the preferred unit of measuring activity as it is the 'natural unit of ambulation'.	If manual step count is considered, the *gold standard*, both the indoor and outdoor accuracy of the SAM is reported as >96% ($n = 18$ healthy subjects). Mean absolute error was reported as 0.5% in 29 subjects, some of whom were post-lower limb surgery, and 0.5% in a sample of 8 who were obese. Accuracy of 99.87% was reported in a sample of healthy able-bodied children, and 97% in a sample of 11 individuals with incomplete spinal cord injury. In a sample of older community-dwelling adults ($n = 34$), the SAM was accurate at all walking speeds and more accurate than the Actigraph accelerometer and the Yamax DigiWalker pedometer. In a sample of older adults ($n = 21$) in assisted living, the SAM was more accurate than the DigiWalker pedometer.	In a sample of people with Parkinson disease ($n = 26$), average physical activity levels (steps per day) were significantly lower in individuals with Hoehn & Yahr stage 3 and higher compared with individuals with Hoehn & Yahr stage 2 or lower. In addition, the mean number of steps/day and mean steps/min in the most active hour correlated with the total UPDRS score, -0.57 and -0.62 respectively. In young men with Duchenne muscular dystrophy (DMD) ($n = 16$) and age-matched healthy individuals, SAM data was significantly lower for the DMD group at 3 different step rates and for total steps taken.	Test–re-test Stroke: chronic ($n = 16$): ICC = 0.97 tested on separate days ($n = 17$): ICC = 0.96 times of testing separated by 48 hours. In a sample of 40 participants >6 months post-stroke, ICCs varied depending on the length of monitoring period – the authors suggest a 3-day monitoring of total step count is most reliable, ICCs range from 0.93–0.99. Incomplete spinal cord injury ($n = 11$): ICC (2,1) = 0.97 for a 10 min walk and 0.99 for a 6 min walk.

Continued

73

Table 8.1 StepWatch™ Monitor – Step Activity Monitor (SAM)—cont'd

Validity			Reliability
Face/content	Criteria validity accuracy	Construct	Relative
	In people post-stroke in the chronic phase ($n = 16$), the SAM is also more accurate than the pedometer. In a sample of participants with stroke ($n = 25$), the criteria used was three dimensional gait analysis (3DGA) and footswitches. Correlations between paretic and non-paretic SAM and 3DGA ranged were 0.90 and 0.95 respectively and >0.97 for footswitches.		

Table 8.2 RT3 accelerometer

Description	User groups	Availability & publications	User-centredness utility
The RT3 accelerometer is a tri-axial accelerometer. Its output can be used to measure activity, intensity of activity and energy expenditure. It is smaller that the original TriTrac accelerometer. It is used in conjunction with a docking station and PC for downloading data captured by the RT3 which is attached to the waist.	Children Healthy adults Overweight and obese adults Stroke Multiple Sclerosis (MS) Parkinson's disease Adults following coronary artery bypass graft (CABG)	www.stayhealthy.com Powell & Rowlands (2004) Rowlands et al (2004) Hertzog et al (2007) Hale et al (2007,2008) Skidmore et al (2008) Jerome et al (2009) Hussey et al (2009) Reneman & Helmus (2009)	In a sample of people with neurological disability ($n = 38$), utility was reported as high, however a sample of people with MS ($n = 10$) reported difficulties with the attachment of the RT3 at the waist were noted.

Validity

Face/content	Criteria validity accuracy
The RT3 accelerometer is a tri-axial accelerometer which captures data in 3 planes.	In a sample of 28 children aged 7–12 years, output of the RT3 used to estimate energy expenditure has been validated against the *gold standard* using an Oxycon mobile system. Correlations between the two methods ranged from 0.56 to 0.84, depending on the activity. In a sample of boys ($n = 19$) correlations between RT3 and steady state oxygen consumption was 0.88 for treadmill tests and 0.82 for unregulated activity. Similar correlations were found for male students ($n = 15$).

Reliability

Relative	Inter-instrument	Absolute
Reliability was evaluated in two trials of 6 activities. 10 min activity data for walking at two speeds, running at two speeds on the treadmill, rest and repeated sit to stand were taken 2 days apart. Reliability between tests 1 and 2 was shown to be good. In a sample of people with neurological disability ($n = 38$): MS, PD, stroke and healthy, sedentary adults ($n = 9$), the reliability of two tests 8 weeks apart was high (ICC 2,1–0.85, 0.74–0.99). There was a significant difference between data gathered over 3 days and 7 days with the latter recommended. In a sample of people with MS, ($n = 10$) RT3 activity data was measured at two time points 1 week apart, ICC (1,1) ranged from 0.50 to 0.76 for various activities.	The data from the trial on reliability was also analysed for inter-instrument or inter-monitor variability; the results indicate that variability existed between the data recorded by 2 RT3s worn at the same time. It varied depending on the activity. It was least for the vertical axis. The ICC for inter-instrument reliability of 6 RT3 monitors worn by 6 healthy subjects doing 3 standardized activities was 0.78, however the lower range for the 95% confidence interval was 0.46 which is low and may be indicative of problems with inter-instrument reliability.	In a sample of people with neurological disability ($n = 38$): MS, PD, stroke and healthy, sedentary adults ($n = 9$), the standard error of the measurement was reported as 23% suggesting that this figure may represent normal fluctuations in PA.

Table 8.3 Physical Activity and Disability Survey (PADS) and Revised Physical Activity and Disability Survey (R-PADS)

Description	Perspective	Language	Availability & publications	User-centredness	Utility
The R-PADS is a revision of the original PADS which is a 6-item scale. The questionnaire asks respondents to report on activity 'last week'. It considers exercise, leisure time physical activity (LTPA), general activity, therapy, employment/school and wheelchair users.	Adults with neurological disability	English	R-PADS is available in Kayes et al (2009) See Appendix 2 Rimmer et al (2001)	It is a self-reported questionnaire developed with input from people with multiple sclerosis who were asked about the acceptability of the questionnaire. Thereafter, it was completed by people with MS and people with stroke and any difficulties expressed were addressed in the revisions.	The scoring is not immediately intuitive but a spreadsheet is available to assist and the instructions are clear.

Validity			Reliability		
Face/content			**Relative**		
Data on 405 subjects with MS and stroke were analysed. Principal component analysis yielded the contributory weight of each item score to the total scores. These weights were incorporated into the calculation of the total score. For ease, a spreadsheet is available for calculation at: http://cre.sagepub.com (Kayes et al 2009).			R-PADS Test–re-test reliability: In a sample of 26 participants whose activity was deemed to be stable between the two tests, ICC (1,1) was reported as 0.91. Bland & Altman limits of agreement were $\pm$ 0.89.		

Table 8.4 Physical Activity Scale for the Elderly (PASE)

Description	Perspective	Language	Availability & publications	User-centredness	Utility
The PASE is a 10-item questionnaire that asks about various activities including household, work, physical activity and exercise in the past 7 days. It records frequency (out of 7 days) and duration (time) and a scoring algorithm is provided with the instruction manual. Preliminary norms are reported.	Older adults: healthy and those with lower extremity disability	English, Japanese	License available to purchase from New England Research Institute's website. It includes administration and scoring manual and up to 200 administrations Washburn et al (1993, 1999) Schuit et al (1997) Martin et al (1999) Dinger et al (2004) Hagiwara et al (2008)	It is a simple to use scale for completion by the user; it asks about activities in the past 7 days. It takes between 5–15 min to complete. It can be administered by interview or completed by the user. It is valid for use by telephone or self-report or by post.	The scoring manual provides coding examples for the activities that may be listed by the user. A computer code is also provided for calculating.

	Validity			Reliability	
Face/content	Criterion including concurrent, predictive and diagnostic		Construct including convergent and discriminant	Relative	

Face/content	Criterion	Construct	Relative
The initial development included a review of the literature and expert opinion and a pilot test with 36 older adults. After the initial development, another iteration was completed by 193 subjects who were also monitored by an accelerometer and completed an activity diary and a global self-report scale. Principal component factor analysis of the three methods of measurement provided the weights assigned to each item. Thereafter, further testing was completed by 222 older adults.	In a sample of 222 older adults, PASE scores correlated with grip strength (0.37), balance (0.33) and overall ratings of perceived health (−0.34). In a sample of 190 older adults PASE scores correlated with peak oxygen uptake (0.20) and balance scores (0.20). In a further study of 21 older adults, scores on a modified PASE for a Dutch population were correlated with the ratio of total energy expenditure and resting metabolic rate (physical activity ratio, PAR) (0.68). In a sample of 20 healthy older adults, PASE scores correlated with 3-day data measured by an accelerometer (0.49).	Expected seasonal variations in physical activity were noted in a sample of 222 older adults, with levels being lower in the winter in New England (correlation with average monthly temperatures − 0.83). The PASE scores of older adults with knee pain ($n = 471$) were examined and those who experience pain more frequently were less physically active.	In a sample of 56 older adults living in a rural area, the PASE was tested on two occasions with very good agreement: ICC = 0.91.

Table 8.5 Stanford 7-Day Physical Activity Recall Questionnaire (7D-PAR) (PAR)

Description	Perspective	Language	Availability & publications	User-centredness	Utility
The 7-day PAR is a semi-structured interview that estimates an individual's time spent in physical activity, strength and flexibility in the 7 days prior to the interview. The day is divided into segments: morning, afternoon and evening. Participants provide information about the amount of time spent in sleep, moderate, hard and very hard activity in bouts >10 min. A recent algorithm (Welk et al 2001) also includes time in sitting. The remainder of the 24 h is deemed to be light. A metabolic equivalent (MET) value is assigned to each level of activity: – Sleep/sitting 1.0 – Light 1.5 – Moderate 4.0 – Hard 6.0 – Very hard 10.0 Physical activity (total energy expenditure) is calculated as kcal/day by multiplying MET × hours × body weight.	Widely used in epidemiological studies for all age groups.	English	Details online, see Kriska (1997) and the Welk algorithm is described in Welk et al (2001) Dishman et al (1988) Hayden-Wade et al (2003) Dubbert et al (2004)	The PAR asks users to recall time spent in sitting, moderate–very hard activity in the past week. Thereafter the interviewer calculates the energy expenditure using a simple algorithm. It can be used in-person or over the telephone.	The online manual provides scoring details and interview instructions. It takes approximately 20 min to complete.

Validity			Reliability	
Face/content	Criterion including concurrent, predictive and diagnostic	Construct including convergent and discriminant	Relative	
The original version of the PAR (PAR1) asked users to account for periods of moderate to very hard activity as it was thought that these are easily recalled. Sleep time was also recalled. The time thereafter, in light activities, was calculated by subtraction. The algorithm used by Welk et al (2001) requires time in sitting to be recalled and included in sleep/rest and removed from light. This addition provides a more valid measure of energy expenditure (PAR2).	Convergent validity of various algorithms used to calculate physical activity and energy expenditure from the PAR is reported by Welk et al (2001) by comparing scores on a TriTrac accelerometer and the two versions of the PAR: PAR1 and PAR2. The PAR scores were significantly correlated with TriTrac activity monitors (0.72), with PAR2 being more accurate (0.77).	Relationships between the PAR and other variables such as a 6-min distance test (0.22), accelerometer readings (0.22/0.23), VO_2max (0.27/0.38) are generally low but are higher with activity logs (0.66–0.71).	Inter-rater reliability in older men ($n = 220$) is high, ranging from ICC of 0.80–0.89 for each of the 4 aspects of the PAR: sleep, moderate, hard and very hard activity and overall estimated energy expenditure. ICCs ranged from 0.58–0.63 for college students ($n = 163$). For children ($n = 46$) ICCs between 2 days were −0.98.	

References

Allor KM, Pivarnik JM: Stability and convergent validity of three physical activity assessments, *Med Sci Sports Exerc* 33(4):671–676, 2001.

Bergman RJ, Bassett DR Jr, Muthukrishman S, et al: Validity of 2 devices for measuring steps taken by older adults in assisted-living facilities, *Journal of Physical Activity and Health* 5(Suppl 1):S166–S175, 2007.

Booth M, Bauman A, Owen N: Physical activity preferences, preferred sources of assistance and perceived barriers to increased activity among physically inactive Australians, *Prev Med* 26:131–137, 1997.

Bowden MG, Behrman AL: Step Activity Monitor: Accuracy and test-re-test reliability in persons with incomplete spinal cord injury, *J Rehabil Res Dev* 44(3):355–362, 2007.

Busse ME, Van Deursen RW, Wiles CM: Real-life step and activity measurement: reliability and validity, *J Med Eng Technol* 33(1):33–41, 2009.

Coleman KL, Smith DG, Boone DA, et al: Step activity monitor: Long-term, continuous recording of ambulatory function, *J Rehabil Res Dev* 36(1):8–18, 1999.

Dinger MK, Oman F, Taylor EL, et al: Stability and convergent validity of the Physical Activity Scale for the Elderly (PASE), *J Sports Med Phys Fitness* 44(2):186–192, 2004.

Dishman RK, Steinhardt M: Reliability and concurrent validity for a 7-d recall of physical activity in college students, *Med Sci Sports Exerc* 20 (1):14–25, 1988.

Dubbert PM, Vander Weg MW, Kirchner KA, et al: Evaluation of the 7-day Physical Activity Recall in Urban and Rural Men, *Med Sci Sports Exerc* 36(9):1646–1654, 2004.

Greenhalgh J, Long AF, Brettle AJ, et al: Reviewing and selecting outcome measures for use in routine practice, *J Eval Clin Pract* 4(4):339–350, 1998.

Haeuber E, Shaughnessy M, Forrester LW, et al: Accelerometer Monitoring of Home- and Community-Based Ambulatory Activity after Stroke, *Arch Phys Med Rehabil* 85:1997–2001, 2004.

Hagiwara A, Ito N, Sawai K, et al: Validity and reliability of the Physical Activity Scale for the Elderly (PASE) in Japanese people, *Geriatr Gerontol Int* 8:143–151, 2008.

Hale LA, Pal J, Becker I: Measuring free-living physical activity in adults with and without neurologic dysfunction with a triaxial accelerometer, *Arch Phys Med Rehabil* 89:1765–1771, 2008.

Hale L, Williams K, Ashton C, et al: Reliability of RT3 accelerometer for measuring mobility in people with multiple sclerosis: Pilot study, *J Rehabil Res Dev* 44(4):619–628, 2007.

Hayden-Wade HA, Coleman KJ, Sallis JF, et al: Validation of the telephone and in-person interview versions of the 7-day PAR, *Med Sci Sports Exerc* 35(5):801–809, 2003.

Hertzog MA, Nieveen JL, Zimmerman LM, et al: Longitudinal field comparison of the RT3 and an activity diary with cardiac patients, *J Nurs Meas* 15(2):105–120, 2007.

Hussey J, Bennett K, O'Dwyer J, et al: Validation of the RT3 in the measurement of physical activity in children, *J Sci Med Sport* 12:130–133, 2009.

Jerome GJ, Young DR, Laferrière D, et al: Reliability of RT3 Accelerometers among overweight and obese adults, *Med Sci Sports Exerc* 41(1):110–114, 2009.

Kayes NM, Schluter PJ, McPherson KM, et al: The physical activity and disability survey – revised (PADS-R): an evaluation of a measure of physical activity in people with chronic neurological conditions, *Clin Rehabil* 23:534–543, 2009.

Kriska AM: A collection of physical activity questionnaires for health-related research – seven-day physical activity recall, *Med Sci Sports Exerc* 29(Suppl 6):S89–S103, 1997.

Macko RF, Haeuber E, Shaughnessy M, et al: Microprocessor-based ambulatory activity monitoring in stroke patients, *Med Sci Sports Exerc* 34(3):394–399, 2002.

Martin KA, Rejeski WJ, Miller ME, et al: Validation of the PASE in older adults with knee pain and physical disability, *Med Sci Sports Exerc* 31(5):627–633, 1999.

McDonald CM, Widman LM, Walsh DD, et al: Use of step activity monitoring for continuous physical activity assessment in boys with Duchenne muscular dystrophy, *Arch Phys Med Rehabil* 86:202–208, 2005a.

McDonald CM, Widman L, Abresch T, et al: Utility of a step activity monitor for the measurement of daily ambulatory activity in children, *Arch Phys Med Rehabil* 86:793–801, 2005b.

Mudge S, Stott SN: Test-re-test reliability of the StepWatch Activity Monitor outputs in individuals with chronic stroke, *Clin Rehabil* 22:871–877, 2008.

Mudge S, Stott S, Walt SE: Criterion validity of the StepWatch Activity Monitor as a measure of walking activity in patients after stroke, *Arch Phys Med Rehabil* 88:1710–1715, 2007.

Powell SM, Rowlands AV: Intermonitor variability of the RT3 Accelerometer during typical physical activities, *Med Sci Sports Exerc* 36(2):324–330, 2004.

Reneman M, Helmus M: Inter-instrument reliability of the RT3 accelerometer, *Int J Rehabil Res* Epub ahead of print, 2009.

Resnick B, Nahm ES, Orwig D, et al: Measurement of activity in older adults: reliability and validity of the Step Activity Monitor, *J Nurs Meas* 9 (3):275–290, 2001.

Rimmer JH, Riley BB, Rublin SS: A new measure for assessing the physical activity behaviours of persons with disabilities and chronic health conditions: The Physical Activity and Disability Survey, *Am J Health Promot* 16(1):34–45, 2001.

Rowlands AV, Thomas PWM, Eston RG, et al: Validation of the RT3 triaxial accelerometer for the assessment of physical activity, *Med Sci Sports Exerc* 36(3):518–524, 2004.

Schuit AJ, Schouten EG, Westerterp KR, et al: Validity of the Physical Activity Scale for the Elderly (PASE): according to energy expenditure assessed by the doubly labeled water method, *J Clin Epidemiol* 50 (5):541–546, 1997.

Shepherd EF, Toloza E, McClung CD, et al: Step Activity Monitor: Increased accuracy in quantifying ambulatory activity, *J Orthop Res* 17:703–708, 1999.

Skidmore FM, Mackman CA, Pav B, et al: Daily ambulatory activity levels in idiopathic Parkinson disease, *J Rehabil Res Dev* 45(9):1343–1348, 2008.

Storti KL, Pettee KK, Bracj JS, et al: Gait speed and step-count monitor accuracy in community-dwelling older adults, *Med Sci Sports Exerc* 40(1):59–64, 2008.

Survey of Lifestyle, Attitudes and Nutrition (SLAN) and The Irish Health Behaviour in School-aged Children Survey (HBSC): *Centre for Health Promotion Studies, National University of Ireland*, Galway, 2006, Department of Health and Children.

Washburn RA, McAuley E, Katula J, et al: The Physical Activity Scale for the Elderly (PASE): Evidence for validity, *J Clin Epidemiol* 52(7):643–651, 1999.

Washburn RA, Smith KW, Jette AM, et al: 1993, The Physical Activity Scale for the Elderly (PASE): Development and Evaluation, 46(2):153–162.

Welk GJ, Thompson RW, Galper DI: A temporal validation of scoring algorithms for the 7-day physical activity recall, *Measurement in Physical Education and Exercise Science* 5(3):123–138, 2001.

Woods C: Exercise and the older person, *Irish Ageing Studies Review* 3(1):11–20, 2009.

Measuring fatigue

9

CHAPTER CONTENTS

Introduction

Fatigue – why is measuring it important? While we have all, no doubt, felt very tired or fatigued from time to time this is usually relieved by a few 'early nights' and restorative sleep. For some individuals, especially those with chronic diseases such as multiple sclerosis (MS), Parkinson's disease, arthritis or chronic obstructive pulmonary disease (COPD), fatigue may an overwhelming symptom (O'Connell & Stokes 2007). It is also well-recognized to be prevalent in people with cancer undergoing radiotherapy and/or chemotherapy (Yamagishi et al 2009, Kim et al 2008). It is reported to be 'grossly under-estimated and misunderstood' (Michael 2002) in conditions such as stroke where it is often thought to be a result of depression; fatigue may occur in the presence of depression but may also exist independent of depression in stroke (Stokes et al 2010).

If individuals taking part in rehabilitation complain of fatigue, then measuring it may be helpful to the patient/client and the therapist in devising home exercise programmes, in planning when exercise and appointments should take place and in some instances, in observing the effect of an intervention on fatigue (McCullagh et al 2008). A variety of methods of measuring fatigue are described in the accompanying Tables and are suitable for use with healthy adults and people with a variety of neurological disabilities and other chronic diseases. The timeframes vary from daily recollections and those covering the past 4 weeks. Some are lengthy and others short and simple to complete.

As described in Chapter 3, the checklist reported by Greenhalgh et al (1998) is the basis for the information provided in the tables that accompany this chapter on each outcome measure. Where relationships between variables are described in the context of validity and reliability, the statistical tests employed are co-efficients such as Pearson Product Moment and Spearman's Rank correlation co-efficient unless otherwise stated. Where details of the exact intra-class correlation (ICC) were provided in the primary source, it is included in the table and if not, the abbreviation ICC is used.

© 2011, Elsevier Ltd.
DOI: 10.1016/B978-0-443-06915-4.00009-7

Table 9.1 Barrow Neurological Institute (BNI) Fatigue Scale

Description	Perspective	Language	Availability & publications	User-centredness	Utility
An 11-item scale, 10 items relating to the extent to which fatigue impacts on the ability to carry out specific activities and one 'overall' fatigue question. Scored from 0 'rarely a problem' to 7 'a problem most of the day'	Acute neurological rehabilitation Self-reported fatigue scale	English	Available in Borgaro et al (2004) See Appendix 3	The focus of the scale is to capture fatigue in individuals who are undergoing neuro-rehabilitation. It was developed because no other extant scales were considered appropriate for this group.	The scale is short and self-reported. It considers tasks that are meaningful for an individual in the acute stage post-brain injury. All 84 participants in the initial study could complete the instrument.

Validity		Reliability	
Face/content	Construct including convergent and discriminant	Relative	Internal consistency
Factor analysis on 84 responses indicates the scale captures one domain explaining 65% of variance.	Construct: the scores on items 1–10 correlated highly with the 'overall' feeling of fatigue since injury (0.671).	Test–re-test ($n = 30$) $= 0.96$	Cronbach's alpha ($n = 84$) $= 0.941$

Table 9.2 Brief Fatigue Inventory

Description	Perspective	Language	Availability & publications	User-centredness	Utility
A 9-item scale. An initial question about feelings of being 'unusually tired in the last week' (Yes/No); 3 items use a numeric rating scale on current fatigue – usual level and worst level in the past 24 h; 6 questions ask how fatigue has interfered with activities in the past 24 h; a numeric rating scale.	Adults with cancer who are outpatients	Originally developed in English. Validated in Korean, Greek, German, Taiwanese, Japanese and Chinese	Available in English in Mendoza et al (1999) See Appendix 3 Wang et al (2004) Okuyama et al (2003) Radbruch et al (2003) Yun et al (2005) Lin et al (2006) Mystakidou et al (2008)	The aim of this scale was to produce a brief measure of fatigue in people with cancer similar to the Brief Pain Inventory, a pain-assessment instrument.	The scale is short and self-reported. It is easily understood for educationally disadvantaged people.

	Validity	

Face/content	Criterion including concurrent, predictive and diagnostic	Construct including convergent and discriminant
The items in the BFI were generated by using the results of a fatigue questionnaire developed by the University of Wisconsin-Madison and completed by both patients and healthy subjects ($n = 249$) as the work of a multi-disciplinary working group. Preliminary analysis of a large sample of both patient and normal subjects less to item reduction.	Discriminant: mean BFI scores were compared across different groups depending on scores on the Eastern Cooperative Oncology Group (ECOG) performance status. Significant differences were noted between different performance status. Concurrent: BFI scores compared with the fatigue subscale of Functional Assessment of Cancer Therapy (FACT) (0.88) and Vigor and Fatigue subscales of Profile of Mood States (POMS) (−0.92).	Construct: Factor analysis on ($n = 578$) responses indicates the scale captures one domain (subjective report of fatigue severity) explaining 75% of the variance.

Table 9.3 Revised Piper Fatigue Scale (R-PFI)

Description	Perspective	Language	Availability & publications	User-centredness	Utility
The original scale described by Piper et al (1989) contained 42 items with anchors of 0–100. The R-PFI contains 22 characteristics of fatigue, with a 0–10 numeric rating scale. There are 5 additional items that provide qualitative information and are not scored.	People with cancer and post-polio. Clark et al (2006) report a review of the R-PFI in caregivers of people with cancer but note that there are some concepts perceived as separate by people with cancer which are not conceptually distinct in their carers.	Originally developed in English. It has also been validated in French (Gledhill et al 2002) and Dutch (Dagnelie et al 2006) for people with cancer.	Available in Piper et al (1998) See Appendix 3 Piper et al (1989) Gledhill et al (2002) Strohschein et al (2003) Clark et al (2006) Ostlund et al (2007) Mota et al (2009)	This scale was designed to be multi-dimensional and to capture fatigue. In its evaluation 4 factors emerged: behaviour/ severity, affective meaning, sensory and cognitive/ mood.	The scale's measurement properties are widely reported in people with cancer. One study has considered people post-polio. It has also been used in studies of people with HIV, myocardial infarction and in pregnancy.

Validity			Reliability		
Face/content	Construct including convergent and discriminant		Relative	Internal consistency	
Cancer: To reduce the initial 43 items to a smaller number, principal axis factor analysis with oblique rotation was performed on a sample of 382 responses from women with breast cancer. In addition, items were excluded if they were gender-specific, Cronbach's alpha of at least 0.89 for items/subscale. Post-polio: 46 post-polio survivors and 23 healthy controls and a team of experts evaluated and agreed that the content of the R-PFI is suitable for measuring fatigue in this population.	Post-polio: Discriminant: Significantly different scores between post-polio subjects and healthy controls. Convergent: The scores of post-polio subjects were strongly correlated with the Chalder Fatigue Questionnaire (0.80).		Post-polio: Test–re-test ($n = 20$) ICC = 0.98	Post-polio ($n = 46$) Cronbach's alpha = 0.98	

Table 9.4 Multi-dimensional Fatigue Inventory (MFI-20)

Description	Perspective	Language	Availability & publications	User-centredness	Utility
A 20-item self-reported instrument that captures 5 dimensions of fatigue: general fatigue, physical fatigue, mental fatigue, reduced motivation and reduced activity. It is scored using a 5-point Likert scale. ≥ 12 on the General Fatigue scale has been reported as an indicator of significant pathological fatigue (Christensen et al 2008).	People with cancer, stroke, and healthy controls	Originally developed in English. It has been validated in French, French Canadian for cancer fatigue and Swedish for people with fibromyalgia and cancer and healthy controls.	French version in Gentile et al (2003), French Canadian in Fillion et al (2003) See Appendix 3 Smets et al (1995) Schneider (1998) Meek et al (2000) Munch et al (2006) Ericsson & Mannerkorpi (2007) Hagelin et al (2007) Christensen et al (2008) Stokes et al (2010)	The scale was originally designed to bridge the gap between one-dimensional fatigue instruments and lengthy multi-dimensional instruments.	It is a self-reported scale which appears to have high acceptability with various groups. Scoring system uses the sum of questions as follows: General fatigue is the sum of questions 1, 5, 12 & 16. Physical fatigue is the sum of questions 2, 8, 14 & 20. Activity is the sum of questions 3, 6, 10 & 17. Motivation is the sum of questions 4, 9, 15 & 18 and mental is the sum of questions 7, 11, 13 & 19.

Validity

Face/content	Construct including convergent and discriminant
Initial item selection was made to include items which would cover 5 postulated domains of fatigue. This first iteration was tested on patients with cancer, and another group with chronic fatigue. A 'healthy' group of students were also included. As well as a group of new junior doctors who were assumed to be 'healthy & fatigued' due to new work experiences & high emotional burden. In addition a group of army recruits were included to capture fatigue due to physical effort. Confirmatory factor analysis was completed and the proposal of a model with 5 domains was supported. 96% of all respondents completed the MFI without omitting items.	Using the various groups, it was hypothesized that fatigue would differ between the groups and convergent validity was tested by comparing MFI-20 scores in patients with cancer and their scores on a 100mm visual analogue scale for fatigue. All 5 sub-scales discriminated between groups. Higher scores were found in patients than in the 'healthy' groups. The relationships between the MFI-20 subscales and the VAS ranged from 0.23–0.77. MFI-20 scores have also been shown to have moderate relationship with the Rhoten fatigue Scale.

Reliability

Internal consistency
Cronbach's alphas vary between groups studied and for each domain. For patients with cancer, alphas were 0.77–0.91, for students, they ranged from 0.76–93 and for army recruits they were lower ranging from 0.53–0.89. In a study of patients with cancer receiving outpatient chemotherapy and/or radiotherapy, alphas ranged from 0.62–0.74.

Table 9.5 Fatigue Severity Scale (FSS)

Description	Perspective	Language	Availability & publications	User-centredness	Utility
The original FSS is a 9-item scale. The user is asked to consider fatigue is the past 2 weeks and each statement is scored on a 7- point Likert scale. A 5-item version has been proposed for MS (Mills et al 2009).	Post-polio, spinal cord injury, Parkinson's disease, multiple sclerosis, systemic lupus erythematosus, chronic hepatitis C	Originally developed in English. It has been validated for use in German, Swedish and Turkish. It has been translated into Australian English, Canadian English and French, French, German, Mexican Spanish, New Zealand English, Spanish, Taiwanese and UK English.	English available in Krupp et al (1989) See Appendix 3 Kleinman et al (2000) Vasconcelos et al (2006) Reske et al (2006) Hagell et al (2006) Armutlu et al (2007) Anton et al (2008) Mattsson et al (2008)	The scale was developed in 1989 to facilitate patient treatment and research.	A short self-reported scale on the impact of fatigue on 8–9 key areas on life.

Validity		Reliability		Measuring change
Criterion including concurrent, predictive and diagnostic	Construct including convergent and discriminant	Relative	Internal consistency	
Factor analysis supports the uni-dimensionality of the 9-item scale in PD and in chronic hepatitis but not in MS. In spinal cord injury (SCI) using a cut-off score of 4, sensitivity and specificity for 'severe fatigue' are 75% and 67%, respectively. In post-polio syndrome, the FSS was more accurate than VAS and Fatigue Impact Scale in identifying subjects with 'disabling fatigue',	Discriminant: FSS discriminated between normal healthy adults, people with MS and systemic lupus erythematosus (SLE). It also discriminated between participants with 'disabling fatigue' and those without in post-polio syndrome. Convergent: In the sample of healthy, MS and SLE, a strong relationship is noted between FSS and VAS scores (0.68). In SCI (0.67), in chronic hepatitis C (0.75), in post-polio syndrome (0.45) for the same comparison.	Test-re-test: SCI ($n = 48$): ICC (1,1) = 0.84 Chronic hepatitis C ($n = 812$): ICC = 0.82	Cronbach's alpha: Normal healthy controls ($n = 20$) = 0.88 MS ($n = 25$) = 0.81 SLE ($n = 29$) = 0.89 SCI ($n = 48$) = 0.89 Chronic hepatitis C ($n = 1223$) = 0.94 PD ($n = 118$) = 0.94	SCI: Standard error of the measurement = 0.55

Table 9.6 Fatigue Impact Scale (FIS) & its derivatives – Daily Fatigue Impact Scale (D-FIS), Modified-Fatigue Impact Scale (M-FIS) and Fatigue Impact Scale for Chronic Obstructive Airways disease (COPD) (FIS-25)

Description	Perspective	Language	Availability & publications	User-centredness	Utility
FIS: 40-item scale measuring the impact of fatigue on cognitive, physical and social functioning. It is scored from 0–4, with 0 'no problem' and 4 'extreme problem'. The scale asks about fatigue in the past month. D-FIS: designed for evaluating the daily impact of fatigue. The 40-item scale is reduced to 8 items. M-FIS: Contains items for people with MS.	FIS: People with MS, chronic fatigue, D-FIS: flu-like illness, Parkinson's disease, MS M-FIS: MS FIS-25: COPD	FIS: French, Swedish M-FIS: English, Italian, Spanish, Slovenian, Flemish FIS-25: English	FIS: Available in Fisk et al (1994) D-FIS: Available in Fisk & Doble (2002) M-FIS: Available online, see references. See Appendix 3 MS Council for Clinical Practice Guidelines, (1998) Mathiowetz (2003) Flachenecker et al (2002) Kos et al (2005) Flensner et al (2005) Martinez-Martin et al (2006) Benito-León et al (2007) Debouverie et al (2007) Theander et al (2007)	The original scale was designed not simply to measure fatigue but to capture its impact on patients' perceptions of functional limitations. The shorter daily version was designed to be a valid and responsive measure of the impact of fatigue on the daily lives of people. Two disease specific versions have also been developed.	Two versions of the original exist – one capturing the impact of fatigue in the past 4 weeks, which has 40 items and considers the multi-dimensional aspect of fatigue. The shorter 8-item version is quick and easy to complete and responsive to daily changes in fatigue.

Validity			Reliability		
Face/content	Criterion including concurrent, predictive and diagnostic	Construct including convergent and discriminant	Relative	Internal consistency	
Initial item selection for the FIS was as a result of a review of existing questionnaires and interviews with 30 people with MS. In addition, the items were tested so that a reading level of $<$Grade 8 would suffice for	D-FIS: Using 'time lost from work' as a criterion, scores on the D-FIS were significantly higher in those in the sample who reported missing work hours compared with those who did not (total sample $n = 93$)	FIS: Discriminant: The FIS was measured in 3 groups – chronic fatigue ($n = 145$), MS ($n = 105$) and mild hypertension ($n = 34$). It was able to discriminate appropriately between the 3 groups.	FIS: Test-re-test: MS ($n = 54$): ICC (3,1) = 0.76 FIS-25: ($n = 143$) – correlation between time 1 and 2, = 0.94 M-FIS: MS ($n = 181$):ICC = 0.99	Cronbach's alpha FIS ($n = 284$) = 0.98 FIS-25 ($n = 296$) = 0.96 M-FIS ($n = 181$) = 0.92 D-FIS ($n = 93$) = 0.91	D-FIS Using the D-FIS is a sample of people with flu-like illness, the D-FIS scores were measured on day 1–5 and on day 10 and day 21 when the subjects were symptom-free. The scores on days 10 and 21 did not differ from one

Continued

Table 9.6 Fatigue Impact Scale (FIS) & its derivatives – Daily Fatigue Impact Scale (D-FIS), Modified-Fatigue Impact Scale (M-FIS) and Fatigue Impact Scale for Chronic Obstructive Airways disease (COPD) (FIS-25)—cont'd

	Validity			Reliability	
Face/content	Criterion including concurrent, predictive and diagnostic	Construct including convergent and discriminant	Relative	Internal consistency	
understanding. A series of Rasch analysis lead to the item reduction for D-FIS. The M-FIS was developed by a panel of experts and people with MS, it is a derived 21-item version (MS Council for Clinical Practice Guidelines 1998). For the development of the FIS-25 in COPD, theory, confirmatory factor analysis and modification indices were used to reduce the items.		Convergent: In a sample of 52 people with MS, the following relationship is noted between FIS and FSS (0.44), FIS and SF-36 Vitality (−0.55), FIS and SF36 Mental Health (−0.62). In 181 people with MS, the relationship between M-FIS and FSS was −0.66. In PD, scores on the D-FIS were correlated with the MFI-General (0.56), MFI-Physical (0.69), MFI-Activity (0.65), MFI-Motivation (0.45) and MFI-Mental (0.60).			another but were significantly different from the other days.

References

Anton H, Miller W, Townson A: Measuring fatigue in persons with spinal cord injury, *Arch Phys Med Rehabil* 89:538–542, 2008.

Armutlu K, Korkmaz N, Keser I, et al: The validity and reliability of the Fatigue Severity Scale in Turkish multiple sclerosis patients, *Int J Rehabil Res* 30:81–85, 2007.

Benito-León J, Martinez-Martin P, Frades B, et al: Impact of fatigue in multiple sclerosis: the Fatigue Impact Scale for Daily Use (D-FIS) *Mult Scler* 13:645–651, 2007.

Borgaro S, Gierok S, Caples H, et al: Fatigue after brain injury: initial reliability study of the B N I Fatigue Scale, *Brain Inj* 18(7):685–690, 2004.

Christensen D, Johnsen S, Watt T, et al: Dimensions of post-stroke fatigue: A two-year follow-up study, *Cerebrovasc Dis* 26:134–141, 2008.

Clark P, Ashford S, Burt R, et al: Factor analysis of the revised piper fatigue scale in a caregiver sample, *J Nurs Meas* 14(2):71–78, 2006.

Dagnelie P, Pijla-Johannesma M, Pijpe A, et al: Psychometric properties of the revised Piper Fatigue Scale in Dutch cancer patients were satisfactory, *J Clin Epidemiol* 59:642–649, 2006.

Debouverie M, Pittion-Vouyovitch S, Louis S, et al: Validity of a French version of the fatigue impact scale in multiple sclerosis, *Mult Scler* 13:1026–1032, 2007.

Ericsson A, Mannerkopi K: Assessment of fatigue in patients with fibromyalgia and chronic widespread pain. Reliability and validity of the Swedish version of the MFI-20, *Disabil Rehabil* 29(22):1665–1670, 2007.

Fillion L, Gélinas C, Simard S, et al: Validation evidence for the French Canadian adaptation of the multidimensional fatigue inventory as a measure of cancer-related fatigue, *Cancer Nurs* 26(2):143–154, 2003.

Fisk J, Doble S: Construction and validation of a fatigue impact scale for daily administration (D-FIS), *Qual Life Res* 11:263–272, 2002.

Fisk J, Ritvo P, Ross L, et al: Measuring the functional impact of fatigue: initial validation of the Fatigue Impact Scale, *Clin Infect Dis* 18(Suppl 1): 79–83, 1994.

Flachenecker P, Kümpfel T, Kallmann B, et al: Fatigue in multiple sclerosis: a comparison of different rating scales and correlation to clinical parameters, *Mult Scler* 8:523–526, 2002.

Flensner G, Ek AC, Söderhamn O: Reliability and validity of the Swedish version of the Fatigue Impact Scale (FIS), *Scand J Occup Ther* 12:170–180, 2005.

Gentile S, Delarozière L, Favre F, et al: Validation of the French 'multidimensional fatigue inventory' (MFI-20), *Eur J Cancer Care (Engl)* 12:58–64, 2003.

Gledhill JA, Rodary C, Mahé C, et al: French validation of the revised Piper Fatigue Scale, *Rech Soins Infirm* 68:50–65, 2002.

Greenhalgh J, Long AF, Brettle AJ, et al: Reviewing and selecting outcome measures for use in routine practice, *J Eval Clin Pract* 4(4):339–350, 1998.

Hagelin C, Wengström Y, Runesdotter S, et al: The psychometric properties of the Swedish Multidimensional Fatigue Inventory MFI-20 in four different populations, *Acta Oncol* 46:97–104, 2007.

Hagell P, Höglund A, Reimer J, et al: Measuring fatigue in Parkinson's Disease: A psychometric study of two brief generic fatigue questionnaires, *J Pain Symptom Manage* 32(5): 420–432, 2006.

Kim SH, Son BH, Hwang SY, et al: Fatigue and depression in disease-free breast cancer survivors: prevalence, correlates, and association with quality of life, *J Pain Symptom Manage* 35(6):644–655, 2008.

Kleinman L, Zodet M, Hakim Z, et al: Psychometric evaluation of the fatigue severity scale for use in chronic hepatitis C, *Qual Life Res* 9:499–508, 2000.

Kos D, Kerckhofs E, Carrea I, et al: Evaluation of the Modified Fatigue Impact Scale in four different European countries, *Mult Scler* 11:76–80, 2005.

Krupp L, LaRocca N, Muir-Nash J, et al: The Fatigue Severity Scale application to patients with multiple sclerosis and systemic lupus erythematosus, *Arch Neurol* 46(10): 1121–1123, 1989.

Lin C, Chang A, Chen M, et al: Validation of the Taiwanese version of the brief fatigue inventory, *J Pain Symptom Manage* 32(1):52–59, 2006.

Martinez-Martin P, Cataln MJ, Benito-León J, et al: Impact of fatigue in Parkinson's disease: The fatigue impact scale for daily use (D-FIS), *Qua Life Res* 15:597–606, 2006.

Mathiowetz V: Test-retest reliability and convergent validity of the fatigue impact scale for persons with multiple sclerosis, *Am J Occup Ther* 57:389–395, 2003.

Mattsson M, Möller B, Lundberg IE, et al: Reliability and validity of the Fatigue Severity Scale in Swedish for patients with systemic lupus erythematosus, *Scand J Rheumatol* 37:269–277, 2008.

McCullagh R, Fitzgerald AP, Murphy RP, et al: Long-term benefits of exercising on quality of life and fatigue in multiple sclerosis patients with mild disability: a pilot study, *Clin Rehabil* 22:206–214, 2008.

Meek P, Nail L, Barsevick A, et al: Psychometric testing of fatigue instruments for use with cancer patients, *Nurs Res* 49(4):181–190, 2000.

Mendoza T, Wang X, Cleeland C, et al: The rapid assessment of fatigue severity in cancer patients, *Cancer* 85:1186–1196, 1999.

Michael K: Fatigue and stroke, *Rehabil Nurs* 27(3):89–103, 2002.

Mills RJ, Young CA, Nicholas RS, et al: Rasch analysis of the Fatigue Severity Scale in multiple sclerosis, *Mult Scler* 15:81–87, 2009.

Mota D, Pimenta C, Piper B: Fatigue in Brazilian cancer patients, caregivers, and nursing students: a psychometric validation study of the Piper Fatigue Scale – Revised, *Support Care Cancer* 17:645–652, 2009.

Multiple Sclerosis Council for Clinical Practice Guidelines: Fatigue and multiple sclerosis: evidence-based management strategies for fatigue in multiple sclerosis, 1998, Multiple Sclerosis Council for Clinical Practice Guidelines Online. Available: http://pva.convio.net/site/News2?page=NewsArticle&id=8101.

Munch TN, Strömgren A, Pedersen L, et al: Multidimensional measurement of fatigue in advanced cancer patients in palliative care: an application of the multidimensional fatigue inventory, *J Pain Symptom Manage* 31(6): 533–541, 2006.

Mystakidou K, Tsilika E, Mendoza T, et al: Psychometric properties of the Brief Fatigue Inventory in Greek patients with advanced cancer, *J Pain Symptom Manage* 36(4):367–373, 2008.

Okuyama T, Wang X, Akechi T, et al: Validation study of the Japanese version of the brief fatigue inventory, *J Pain Symptom Manage* 25 (2):106–117, 2003.

Ostlund U, Gustavsson P, Fürst CJ: Translation and cultural adaptation of the Piper Fatigue Scale for use in Sweden, *Eur J Oncol Nurs* 11:133–140, 2007.

O'Connell C, Stokes EK: Fatigue-concepts for physiotherapy management and measurement, *Phys Ther Rev* 12:314–323, 2007.

Piper BF, Dibble SL, Dodd MJ, et al: The revised Piper Fatigue Scale: psychometric evaluation in women with breast cancer, *Oncol Nurs Forum* 25(4):677–684, 1998.

Piper BF, Lindsey AM, Dodd MJ, et al: The development of an instrument to measure the subjective dimension of fatigue. In Funk SG, Tornquist EM, Champagne MT, et al., editors: *Key aspects of comfort: management of pain, fatigue and nausea*, New York, 1989, Springer, pp 199–208.

Radbruch L, Sabatowski R, Elsner F, et al: Validation of the German version of the brief fatigue inventory, *J Pain Symptom Manage* 25(5):449–458, 2003.

Reske D, Pukrop R, Scheinig K, et al: Measuring fatigue in patients with multiple sclerosis with standardized methods in German speaking areas, *Fortschr Neurol Psychiatr* 74(9): 497–502, 2006.

Schneider R: Reliability and validity of the multidimensional fatigue inventory (MFI-20) and the Rhoten Fatigue Scale among rural cancer outpatients, *Cancer Nurs* 21(5): 370–373, 1998.

Smets E, Garsen B, Bonke B, et al: The multidimensional fatigue inventory (MFI). Psychometric qualities of an instrument to assess fatigue, *Journal of Psychometric Research* 39(5): 315–325, 1995.

Stokes EK, Murphy B, O'Connell C: An investigation into fatigue post stroke and its multidimensional nature (in press), 2010.

Strohschein FJ, Kelly CG, Clarke AG, et al: Applicability, validity and reliability of the Piper Fatigue Scale in postpolio patients, *Am J Phys Med Rehabil* 82(2):122–129, 2003.

Theander K, Cliffordson C, Torstensson O, et al: Fatigue Impact Scale: Its validation in patients with chronic obstructive pulmonary disease, *Psychol Health Med* 12(4): 470–484, 2007.

Vasconcelos O, Prokhorenko O, Kelley K, et al: A comparison of Fatigue Scales in post-poliomyelitis syndrome, *Archives of Medicine and Rehabilitation* 87:1213–1217, 2006.

Wang X, Hao X, Wang Y, et al: Validation study of the Chinese version of the brief fatigue inventory (BFI-C), *J Pain Symptom Manage* 27(4): 322–332, 2004.

Yamagishi A, Morita T, Miyashita M, et al: Symptom prevalence and longitudinal follow-up in cancer outpatients receiving chemotherapy, *J Pain Symptom Manage* 37(5): 823–830, 2009.

Yun Y, Wang X, Lee J, et al: Validation study of the Korean version of the Brief Fatigue Inventory, *J Pain Symptom Manage* 29(2):165–172, 2005.

Measuring neurological conditions and rehabilitation

CHAPTER CONTENTS

Introduction

This chapter contains the review of a number of measurement instruments for use with people with stroke, multiple sclerosis (MS) and Parkinson's disease (PD). Instruments such as these are often described as disease-specific measures and are reported to be under-utilized in clinical practice compared with generic measures (Stokes & O'Neill 1999, 2009).

A number of the instruments included are multi-dimensional, such as the Multiple Sclerosis Impact Scale, the Stroke Impact Scale and SCOPA/SPES and certain domains within each measure may be

of use in your clinical practice rather that the full instrument. As with a number of the fatigue scales, shorter versions have been designed and evaluated, e.g. the SIS-16, which has its focus on physical function. The Motor Assessment Scale is also multidimensional but its focus is on motor function rather than including other domains such as memory, mood and participation.

Two scales take a more focused look at postural stability and trunk impairment – common sources of problem solving and evaluation during rehabilitation. And the Freezing of Gait Questionnaire considers a common problem in people with Parkinson's disease.

Neurological disability is a frequent cause for presentation for rehabilitation; the opinion of the person with the condition and the carers is of vital importance, hence the inclusion of self-reported scales balanced with those that require the observation of performance.

As described in Chapter 3, the checklist reported by Greenhalgh et al (1998) is the basis for the information provided in the tables that accompany this chapter on each outcome measure. Where relationships between variables are described in the context of validity and reliability, the statistical tests employed are co-efficients such as Pearson Product Moment and Spearman's Rank correlation co-efficient unless otherwise stated. Where details of the exact intra-class correlation (ICC) were provided in the primary source, it is included in the table and if not, the abbreviation ICC is used.

DOI: 10.1016/B978-0-443-06915-4.00010-3

Table 10.1 Scales for Outcomes in Parkinson's Disease (SCOPA) – Short Parkinson's Evaluation Scale (SPES)

Description	Perspective	Language	Availability & publications	User-centredness	Utility
The Unified Parkinson's Disease Rating Scale (UPDRS) is a widely known scale for use with people with Parkinson's Disease (PD). The SPES/SCOPA is a derivative of the UPDRS modified to be shortened and to have acceptable measurement properties. It contains 3 sub-sections: Motor Evaluation (ME), Activities of Daily Living (ADL) and Motor complications. A total of 21 items are scored from 0–3.	Parkinson's disease	English, Spanish	Available in Marinus et al (2004) See Appendix 4 Fahn et al (1987) van Hilten et al (1994) Rabey et al (1997) Martignoni et al (2003) Martinez-Martin et al (2005)	The scale is a mix of observation and self-reporting on the part of the individual with PD.	The original UPDRS took approximately 15–20 min to complete, the SPES/SCOPA takes approximately 8 min

Validity			Reliability		
Face/content	Criterion including concurrent, predictive and diagnostic	Construct including convergent and discriminant	Relative	Absolute	Internal consistency
Item reduction from UPDRS was initially reported by van Hilten et al (1994) in 111 subjects with PD. The ADL and	Spanish SPES/SCOPA Concurrent validity: SPES/SCOPA scores were strongly correlated with UPDRS scores (>0.7)	English SPES/SCOPA Construct: In a sample of 85 people with PD, SPES/SCOPA sections correlated with	English SPES/SCOPA Inter-rater clinical assessments ($n = 33$ subjects)	Spanish SPES/SCOPA SEM Motor Evaluation (ME) = 2.5 SEM Activities of Daily Living (ADL) = 1.2	English SPES/SCOPA Cronbach's alpha ($n = 85$) = 0.74–0.95 Spanish SPES/SCOPA

ME sections were reduced to 8 items each using principal component factor analysis. Thereafter the SPES was proposed removing items from the UPDRS which were 'considered difficult to evaluate, redundant, or of minor clinical significance. The SPES/SCOPA is a further modification of the SPES to improve the scale construction. Forwards–backwards translation for Spanish version has been completed.

related sections in UPDRS (0.88–0.95).
Discriminant: Participants grouped by Hoehn & Yahr stages had significantly different scores between stages 2, 4 and 3, 4.

Strength of agreement reported as 'moderate' for all items except 'postural tremor right hand' and 'rigidity right hand' which were fair.
$ICC = 0.58$ (0.50 for UPDRS)

SEM
Motor complications $= 0.4$

Cronbach's alpha
($n = 151$)
$= 0.91$–0.95

Table 10.2 Freezing of Gait Questionnaire (FOG-Q) and New Freezing of Gait Questionnaire (NFOG-Q)

Description	Perspective	Language	Availability & publications	User-centredness	Utility
FOG-Q is a 6-item scale which captures self-reported freezing of gait. It is scored on a 0–4 item scale. The New Freezing of Gait Questionnaire is a further development of the FOG. A video may be used and the scale has 8 items.	Parkinson's disease	English, Swedish	FOG-Q available in Giladi et al (2000) NFOG-Q available in Nieuwboer et al (2009) See Appendix 4	The FOG-Q and NFOG-Q are self-reported scales which ask users to report on frequency, duration and impact of freezing. Reports by carers have good agreement with those of people with PD and so may be used as a proxy.	Short, easy to use scale. The NFOG-Q includes a video and considers both FOG severity and impact on daily life. It is not recommended to use the video in clinical practice but it may be helpful for research purposes.

Validity			**Reliability**	
Face/content	Criterion including concurrent, predictive and diagnostic	Construct including convergent and discriminant	Relative	Internal consistency
An initial version tested on 40 participants included 16 items which were reduced to 10 after principal component factor analysis with varimax rotation. Thereafter a 6-item version was chosen based on item-total score correlations and medical considerations. Further testing on a sample of 454 subjects with principal component factor analysis indicated one factor accounting for 64.7% of the variance. Factor analysis of the NFOG-Q yielded two components accounting for 65% of variance – all items loaded equally on main component.	FOG-Q Concurrent: Scores correlated with UPDRS as follows: UPDRS total (0.48) UPDRS ADL (0.43) UPDRS ME (0.40) and with Hoehn & Yahr (0.66). FOG-Q scores correlated highly with UPDRS FOG scores (0.77). Similar relationships are noted in the Swedish version of the FOG-Q (n = 37)	FOG-Q Convergent and divergent: In a large sample (n = 454), scores on the FOG were better correlated with UPDRS sections conceptually related to FOG and less with those that were not, e.g. mental function and depression	FOG-Q Test-re-test: Comparison between baseline and 10 weeks later in a placebo group (part of a larger trial) – correlation of scores = 0.83 NFOG-Q In a sample of 69 people with PD and their carers, agreement was highly satisfactory, ICC (1,1) = 0.75–0.78.	FOG-Q Cronbach's alpha (n = 40) = 0.94; (n = 454) = 0.89. All items contribute to internal consistency, i.e. removal of any item reduces the alpha. NFOG-Q Cronbach's alpha = 0.84

Table 10.3 Postural Assessment Scale for Stroke (PASS)

Description	Perspective	Language	Availability & publications	User-centredness	Utility
The original PASS is a scale for evaluating postural stability after stroke with two components i.e. maintaining a posture and changing posture; it has a total of 17 items and is scored 0–3 on each activity. The scoring is reduced to 3 levels in the (PASS-3L), i.e. 0–1.5–3 and to 5 items in the Short form (SFPASS).	Stroke	English	PASS available in Benaim et al (1999); PASS-3L available in Wang et al (2004); SFPASS available in Chien et al (2007b) See Appendix 4 Mao et al (2002) Chien et al (2007a,b) Liaw et al (2008)	The PASS and its derivatives require the observation of the patient's performance.	The original PASS was reported to take 10 min to perform. The derivatives were designed to make this time shorted.

Validity			Reliability			Measuring Change
Face/content	Criterion including concurrent, predictive and diagnostic	Construct including convergent and discriminant	Relative	Absolute	Internal consistency	
The item inclusion within the scale aimed to capture both static and dynamic postural control; the designers believed that the scale should be suitable for all levels of postural control and it should contain items of increasing levels of difficulty. The original version was adopted from items included	PASS Predictive: PASS scores on 30 days after stroke (DAS) was strongly related (0.75) to scores on the Functional Independence Measure (FIM) on 90 DAS (n = 70). In another sample (n = 101) PASS scores on 14, 30 and 90 DAS were highly correlated with scores on Motor Assessment Scale (MAS) (≥0.80).	PASS Convergent: PASS scores (n = 101) on 14, 30, 60, 90 DAS highly correlated with BI (≥0.86). In initial development (n = 70), PASS scores correlated highly with FIM (0.78) and lower limb motoricity (0.78). Discriminant: In a sample of age-matched healthy adults (n = 30), all but 3 of the controls scored full marks.	PASS Inter-rater: (n = 12) Bland & Altman plots reveal very good agreement between raters. (n = 101) ICC = 0.97. Test-re-test in chronic stage (>6 months) (n = 52) ICC (2,1) 0.97.	PASS MDC_{95} in a sample of stroke in chronic stage (>6 months) = 3.16 SFPASS (n = 287 acute phase) SEM = 3.4 Suggesting that MDC_{95} could be close to 9.	PASS Cronbach's alpha = 0.95 (n = 70), = 0.94 on 14, 30, 60, 90 DAS (n = 101) SFPASS-3L Cronbach's alpha (n = 287) = 0.93.	PASS Effect size (n = 101) 14–30 DAS = 0.89, 30–90 DAS = 0.64 PASS-3L SRM was best for change between 14 and 30 DAS = 0.86.

Continued

97

Table 10.3 Postural Assessment Scale for Stroke (PASS)—cont'd

Validity			Reliability			Measuring Change
Face/content	Criterion including concurrent, predictive and diagnostic	Construct including convergent and discriminant	Relative	Absolute	Internal consistency	
with the Fugl-Meyer assessment. The PASS-3L and the SFPASS were developed to produce a shorter version of the PASS.	Concurrent: PASS scores on 14, 30, 90, 180 DAS (n = 101) strongly correlated with Berg balance Scale (BBS) (0.92–0.95) and Barthel Index (BI) (0.95–0.97). PASS-3L Concurrent: (n = 77) Score on the PASS-3L were compared with scores on the PASS using the Bland & Altman plots and ICC [1,1]. All but 3 observations feel outside ± 2 SD, ICC = 0.97. Predictive: (n = 226) Score on PASS-3L on 14 and 30 DAS were compared with scores on BI at 90 DAS (0.82).	Single leg leg stance caused the lower score in normals. PASS-3L Convergent: PASS-3L & BI (n = 77) were compared with a strong relationship reported (0.94).				

Table 10.4 Trunk Impairment Scale (TIS)

Description	Perspective	Language	Availability & publications	User-centredness	Utility
A scale to evaluate motor impairment in the truck, containing 3 sections and scored from 0–23. Section 1 addresses sitting balance; section 2 considers dynamic sitting balance and section 3 deals with coordination.	Stroke MS Parkinson's disease Traumatic Brain Injury (TBI)	English	Available in Verheyden et al (2004) See Appendix 4 Verheyden et al (2004, 2005, 2006a, 2006b, 2007)	The TIS requires observation of the response of the patient to a series of instructions or manoeuvres conducted by the assessor. Originally designed for use in people with stroke.	This is a short observational scale (10 min). It is carried out with the patient sitting on a treatment couch or bed; one item is timed.

Validity		Reliability	
Criterion including concurrent, predictive and diagnostic	Construct including convergent and discriminant	Relative	Absolute
Concurrent: Stroke (n = 30) TIS and Trunk Control Test relationship was strong (0.83). In MS (n = 30) scores in TIS were correlated with FIM (0.81) and Extended Disability Status Scale (EDSS) (−0.85). In TBI, scores on TIS correlated with the Barthel Index (BI).	Stroke (n = 30): Construct: TIS and BI correlation (−0.83) Discriminant: Stroke (n = 40) compared with 40 age and gender-matched healthy adults, significant differences in scores were noted, with 55% of the sample obtaining maximum scores. In PD (n = 26). Construct: Those with PD in the early stages had significantly lower scores than participants in the later stages (H&Y stages 4 & 5) of the disease. Correlations with UPDRS Part III (−0.68), UPDRS turning in bed (−0.48), FOG-Q (−0.21). Discriminant: Age and gender-matched healthy adults had significantly higher scores.	Stroke (n = 28): Inter-rater % agreement ranged from 82–100% with Kappa and wKappa values from 0.70–1 and ICC = 0.99. Test-re-test: % agreement ranged from 82–100% with Kappa and wKappa values from 0.46–1 and ICC = 0.96. MS (n = 30): Inter-rater % agreement ranged from 70–100% with Kappa and wKappa values from 0.46–1 and ICC (2,1) = 0.97. Test-re-test: % agreement ranged from 73–100% with Kappa and wKappa values from 0.49–1 and ICC (2,1) = 0.95. TBI: Test-re-test (n = 30) ICC = 0.72. Inter-rater (n = 30) ICC = 0.88.	In MS, the standard error of the measurement is reported as 1.6.

Table 10.5 Multiple Sclerosis Impact Scale (MSIS-29)

Description	Perspective	Language	Availability & publications	User-centredness	Utility
A 29-item scale with two subsections – physical impact and psychological impact. Each item is scored from 1–5 on a Likert scale with anchors 'not at all' and 'extremely'. The most recent iteration is MSIS-29 v2.	MS	English	Available in Hobart et al (2001) See Appendix 4 Riazi et al (2002) Riazi et al (2003) Hobart et al (2004, 2005) van der Linden et al (2005) Giordano et al (2009) Gray et al (2009) Hobart & Cano (2009)	The MSIS-29 was developed following interviews with 30 people with MS. The resultant scale is self-reported and asks about impact in the past 2 weeks. It has been validated for use in a postal survey, in community and hospital (in and outpatient) based samples. It has been validated for use in people with MS receiving rehabilitation, admitted for intravenous corticosteroid treatment for relapses and people with primary progressive MS.	The scores for the two subsections are reported separately. They are simple to complete. It has been shown to have test-re-test reliability when completed by proxies but the relationship between self-reported scores and proxy scores has not been investigated.

Validity		Reliability		Measuring change
Face/content	Construct including convergent and discriminant	Relative	Internal consistency	
Initial item generation was from interviews with 30 people with MS, expert opinion and a review of the literature; 129 items reviewed; and a postal survey to 1500 members of the MS Society in the UK. Analysis of the returned questionnaires (n = 766) yielded a 29-item instrument with two subscales. Initial evaluation on this scale, the MSIS-29 v. 1. Recent Rasch analysis (Hobart & Cano 2009) has 'detected	MSIS-29 Physical subscale Convergent validity: Inpatients (n = 121) correlated with SF-36 physical functioning (−0.63) and FAMS mobility (−0.71). Discriminant validity: In the same sample, weak relationships between physical subscale and measures of mental health and emotional well-being. MSIS Psychological subscale	Test-re-test: In a postal sample (n = 128) Physical impact ICC = 0.94, Psychological impact ICC = 0.87 Reliability has been reported in a sample of people who completed the scale by proxy.	Cronbach's alpha In a postal sample (n = 703) Physical impact = 0.96 Psychologicali Impact = 0.87 In a community sample (n = 248) Physical impact = 0.97 and Psychological impact = 0.93	Initial data on a sample (n = 55) after rehabilitation and IV steroids yielded effect sizes of 0.82 (physical impact) and 0.66 (psychological impact) and in a similar sample (n = 104) standardized response means of 0.58 and 0.45, respectively. When compared with other measures of physical functioning (n = 245, rehabilitation, IV steroids and PMS), the MSIS-29 physical impact was most

important limitations of the MSIS-29 which were not identified by traditional psychometric methods'; this has resulted in a new version with 12 items – MSIS-29 v.2 which is currently being evaluated.

Convergent validity:
Inpatients ($n = 121$)
Correlated with SF-36 mental health (-0.75) and FAMS emotional health (-0.70).
Discriminant validity:
In the same sample, weak relationships between psychological subscale and measures of physical health and mobility.
These relationships are replicated in studies including participants who are inpatients receiving rehabilitation, treatment with corticosteroids. Also replicated across groups with primary progressive, relapsing and remitting and secondary progressive MS.

responsive and MSIS-29 psychological impact was second to the General Health Questionnaire-12.
Using patient reported global measures of change ($n = 104$), the area under the ROC was 0.68 for the physical impact better than FAMS and MSQOL physical health components and 0.65 for the psychological impact better than FAMS and similar to MSQOL mental health components.

Table 10.6 Stroke Impact Scale

Description	Perspective	Language	Availability & publications	User-centredness	Utility
The SIS version 3 (v3.0) has 8 domains which consider physical problems: memory/ thinking, mood, communication, activities, mobility, hand function and participation, which are scored on a 5-point Likert scale. A final section is an estimation of the overall recovery after stroke. SIS-16 has 16 items and focuses on physical ability in the past 2 weeks.	Stroke	Website in reference list provides a list of all languages into which the SIS v. 3.0 and SIS-16 and proxy versions have been translated (see PROQOLID).	Available online & see Appendix 4. Reliability and validity are reported in Dutch, German, English-Australian (version 2.0) and Brazilian (version 3) Duncan et al (1999, 2003) Edwards & O'Connell (2003) Kwon et al (2006) Carod-Artal et al (2008) Geyh et al (2009)	The development of the SIS involved people with stroke, carers, and experts in stroke. To complete the SIS, an individual must have a score on the mini-mental state examination of >16.	The impact of stroke and the extent of recovery are evaluated in SIS version 3 and the timeframe is in the past week. The SIS-16 item asks about the past 2 weeks. Instructions for use are available online.

Validity		Reliability		Measuring change
Face/content	Construct including convergent and discriminant	Relative	Internal consistency	
	Construct: SIS v. 3.0 Rasch analysis (n = 696) demonstrated that each domain is unidimensional – with the mobility, hand function, participation and physical being very robust from a measurement property perspective. SIS v. 2.0 by telephone	SIS version 2 (n = 25) ICCs for 8 domains = 0.7–0.92	SIS version 2 (n = 91) Cronbach's alpha = 0.83–0.90	SIS version 2 Responsiveness to change over the course of time post-stroke is reported to be informed by severity. For minor strokes: SIS is sensitive to change from 1–3 and 1–6 months but not 3–6 for hand function,

The SIS version 2 (v 2.0) was initially evaluated in 91 people post-stroke and was further evaluated using Rasch analysis in a large sample (n = 696). The analysis resulted in changes and the production of the SIS version 3.0.

Five items were deleted. The physical domain was shown to be the most useful in capturing a range of ability and from this the SIS-16 was developed.

In a sample of people with stroke who completed the SIS v. 2.0 by telephone ($n = 95$) 12 weeks after discharge, correlations with FIM scores at 16 weeks were appropriate, e.g. FIM Motor and SIS Physical composite (0.77), Mobility (0.73), ADL (0.85).
Discriminant:
SIS v. 2.0
The 6/8 SIS domains were able to discriminate between 4 groups within the sample base on Modified Rankin Scores.

ADL, composite physical and participation. For moderate strokes: sensitive to change from 1–3 and 1–6 months and for mobility, ADL, composite physical and participation domains responsive 3–6 months.

Table 10.7 Motor Assessment Scale

Description	Perspective	Language	Availability & publications	User-centredness	Utility
Originally a 9-item scale but modified to an 8-item scale by excluding an item on tone Measured using ordinal scale 0–7.	Stroke	English, Norwegian	Available in Carr et al (1985) Revised upper limb items in Sabari et al (2005) See Appendix 4 Loewen & Anderson (1988) Dean & Mackey (1992) Malouin et al (1994) Poole & Whitney (1998) Hsueh & Hsieh (2002) Johnson & Selfe (2004) Lannin (2004) Kjendahl et al (2005) English & Hillier (2006)	Assessor observes performance on everyday motor activities.	15–17 min to administer. Easy and only simple equipment needed. Practice on 6 patients for training.

	Validity		Reliability		Measuring change
Face/content	Criterion including concurrent, predictive and diagnostic	Relative	Internal consistency		

Face/content	Criterion including concurrent, predictive and diagnostic	Relative	Internal consistency	Measuring change
The initial version included an item on tone but this was removed in later studies. In one early study, an issue with scoring on advanced hand activities was reported. Later, research using Rasch analysis on the 3 upper-limb sections of MAS supported the hierarchical structure of the upper arm function but suggested changes were needed to hand movements and advanced hand activities (see Sabari et al 2005). The scoring is not hierarchical in this section; hence the number of successful tasks completed represents the score. A floor (walking) and ceiling (lying to sitting, balanced sitting, sit to stand and walking) effect has been noted ($n = 61$, inpatients).	Concurrent: ($n = 30$) correlation of 0.88 without tone with Fugl-Meyer (0.5–96 months after stroke) ($n = 32$) acute phase correlation of 0.96 with FM	Inter-rater: Preliminary reports on inter-rater: 87% agreement with criterion rating of performance and 78–95% between raters (5 subjects, 5 therapists). Replicated later but with the removal of tone item in two studies ($n = 24$, $n = 5$). Across all levels of experience. Test–re-test ($n = 15$, 1 rater) also good. Replicated later in a study ($n = 5$) without tone item.	Cronbach's alpha ($n = 26$, acute phase) $= 0.94$	Effect sizes measured in a sample of 61 inpatients ranged from 0.61 to 1.03 for all items except the 3 upper limb items which had low effect sizes. The results for the upper limb items are replicated in another study of 48 inpatients.

References

Benaim C, Pérennou DA, Villy J, et al: Validation of a standardized assessment of postural control in stroke patients, *Stroke* 30:1862–1868, 1999.

Carod-Artal FJ, Coral LF, Trizotto DS, et al: The stroke impact scale 3.0: evaluation of acceptability, reliability, and validity of the Brazilian version, *Stroke* 39:2477–2484, 2008.

Carr JH, Shepherd RB, Nordholm L, et al: Investigation of a new motor assessment scale for stroke patients, *Phys Ther* 65:175–180, 1985.

Chien C, Hu M, Tang P, et al: A comparison of psychometric properties of the smart balance master system and the postural assessment scale for stroke in people who have had mild stroke, *Arch Phys Med Rehabil* 88:374–380, 2007a.

Chien C, Lin J, Wang C, et al: Developing a short form of the postural assessment scale for people with stroke, *Neurorehabil Neural Repair* 21:81–90, 2007b.

Dean C, Mackey F: Motor Assessment Scale scores as a measure of rehabilitation outcome following stroke, *Australian Physiotherapy* 38:31–35, 1992.

Duncan PW, Bode RK, Min Lai S, et al: Rasch analysis of a new stroke-specific outcome scale: the stroke impact scale, *Arch Phys Med Rehabil* 84:950–963, 2003.

Duncan PW, Lai SM, Bode RK, et al: The stroke impact scale version 2.0: evaluation of reliability, validity, and sensitivity to change, *Stroke* 20:2131–2140, 1999.

Edwards B, O'Connell B: Internal consistency and validity of the Stroke Impact Scale 2.0 (SIS 2.0) and SIS-16 in an Australian sample, *Qua Life Res* 12:1127–1135, 2003.

English CK, Hillier SL: The sensitivity of three commonly used outcome measures to detect change amongst patients receiving inpatient rehabilitation following stroke, *Clin Rehabil* 20:52–55, 2006.

Fahn S, Elton RL: Unified Parkinson's disease rating scale. In Fahn S, Marsden CD, Calne D, Goldstein M, editors: *Recent developments in Parkinson's disease*, Florham Park, NJ, 1987, Macmillan Health Care Information, pp 153–164.

Geyh S, Cieza A, Stucki G: Evaluation of the German translation of the Stroke Impact Scale using Rasch analysis, *Clin Neuropsychol* 23(6):978–995, 2009.

Giladi N, Tal J, Azulay T, et al: Validation of the freezing of gait questionnaire in patients with Parkinson's disease, *Mov Disord* 24:655–661, 2009.

Giladi N, Shabtai H, Simon ES, et al: Construction of freezing of gait questionnaire for patients with Parkinsonism, *Parkinsonism Relat Disord* 6:165–170, 2000.

Giordano A, Pucci E, Naldi P, et al: Responsiveness of patient-reported outcome measures in multiple sclerosis relapses: the REMS study, *J Neurol Neurosurg Psychiatry* 80:1023–1028, 2009.

Gray OM, McDonnell GV, Hawkins SA: Tried and tested: the psychometric properties of the multiple sclerosis impact scale (MSIS-29) in a population-based study, *Mult Scler* 15:75–80, 2009.

Greenhalgh J, Long AF, Brettle AJ, et al: Reviewing and selecting outcome measures for use in routine practice, *J Eval Clin Pract* 4(4):339–350, 1998.

Hobart JC, Cano S: Improving the evaluation of therapeutic interventions in multiple sclerosis: the role of new psychometric methods, *Health Technol Assess* 13(iii), ix–x, 1–177, 2009.

Hobart JC, Riazi A, Lamping DL, et al: How responsive is the Multiple Sclerosis Impact Scale (MSIS-29)? A comparison with some other self report scales, *J Neurol Neurosurg Psychiatry* 76:1539–1543, 2005.

Hobart JC, Riazi A, Lamping DL, et al: Improving the evaluation of therapeutic interventions in multiple sclerosis: development of a patient-based measure of outcome, *Health Technol Assess* 8(iii):1–48, 2004.

Hobart JC, Lamping D, Fitzpatrick R, et al: The Multiple Sclerosis Impact Scale (MSIS-29) A new patient-based outcome measure, *Brain* 124:962–973, 2001.

Hsueh IP, Hsieh CL: Responsiveness of two upper extremity function instruments for stroke inpatients receiving rehabilitation, *Clin Rehabil* 16:617–624, 2002.

Johnson L, Selfe J: Measurement of mobility following stroke: a comparison of the Modified Rivermead Mobility Index and the Motor Assessment Scale, *Physiotherapy* 90:132–138, 2004.

Kjendahl A, Jahnsen R, Aamodt G: Motor assessment scale in Norway: Translation and inter-rater reliability, *Advances in Physiotherapy* 7:7–12, 2005.

Kwon S, Duncan P, Studenski S, et al: Measuring stroke impact with SIS: Construct validity of S I S telephone administration, *Qual Life Res* 15:367–376, 2006.

Lannin NA: Reliability, validity and factor structure of the upper limb subscale of the Motor Assessment Scale (UL-MAS) in adults following stroke, *Disabil Rehabil* 26:109–115, 2004.

Liaw L, Hsieh C, Lo S, et al: The relative and absolute reliability of two balance performance measures in chronic stroke patients, *Disabil Rehabil* 30:656–661, 2008.

Loewen SC, Anderson BA: Reliability of the Modified Motor Assessment Scale and the Barthel Index, *Phys Ther* 68:1077–1081, 1988.

Malouin F, Pichard L, Bonneau C, et al: Evaluating Motor Recovery early after stroke: Comparison of the Fugl-Meyer Assessment and the Motor Assessment Scale, *Arch Phys Med Rehabil* 75:1206–1212, 1994.

Mao HF, Hseuh I, Tang P, et al: Analysis and comparison of the psychometric properties of three balance measures for stroke patients, *Stroke* 33:1022–1027, 2002.

Marinus J, Visser M, Stiggelbout AM, et al: A short scale for the assessment of motor impairments and disabilities in Parkinson's disease: the SPES/SCOPA, *J Neurol Neurosurg Psychiatry* 75:388–395, 2004.

Martignoni E, Franchignoni F, Pasetti C, et al: Psychometric properties of the Unified Parkinson's Disease Rating Scale and of the Short Parkinson's Evaluation Scale, *Neurol Sci* 24:190–191, 2003.

Martinez-Martin P, Benito-León J, Burguera JA, et al: The SCOPA-

Motor Scale for assessment of Parkinson's disease is a consistent and valid measure, *J Clin Epidemiol* 58:674–679, 2005.

Nieuwboer A, Rochester L, Herman T, et al: The new Freezing of Gait Questionnaire: ratings from patients with Parkinson's disease and their carers, *Gait Posture* 30:459–463, 2009.

Nieuwboer A, Giladi N: The challenge of evaluating freezing of gait in patients with Parkinson's disease, *Br J Neurosurg* 22(Suppl 1):S16–S18, 2008.

Nieuwboer A, Herman T, Rochester L, et al: The new revised freezing of gait questionnaire, a reliable and valid instrument to measure freezing in Parkinson's disease? *Parkinsonism Relat Disord* 14 (Suppl 1):568, 2008.

Nilsson MH, Hagell P: Freezing of Gait Questionnaire: validity and reliability of the Swedish version, *Acta Neurol Scand* 19 May [Epub ahead of print] 2009.

Poole JL, Whitney SL: Motor assessment scale for stroke patients: concurrent validity and interrater reliability, *Arch Phys Med Rehabil* 69:195–197, 1988.

PROQOLID: *Patient reported outcome and quality of life database*, 2009. Online Available: www.proqolid.org/instruments/stroke_impact_scale_stroke_toolbox_sis Accessed July 22, 2009.

Rabey JM, Bass H, Bonuccelli U, et al: Evaluation of the Short Parkinson's Evaluation Scale: a new friendly scale for the evaluation of Parkinson's disease in clinical drug trials, *Clin Neuropharmacol* 20:322–337, 1997.

Riazi A, Hobart JC, Lamping DL, et al: Evidence-based measurement in multiple sclerosis: the psychometric properties of the physical and psychological dimensions of three quality of life rating scales, *Mult Scler* 9:411–419, 2003.

Riazi A, Hobart JC, Lamping DL, et al: Multiple Sclerosis Impact Scale (MSIS-29): reliability and validity in hospital based samples, *J Neurol Neurosurg Psychiatry* 73:701–704, 2002.

Sabari JS, Lim AL, Velozo CA, et al: Assessing arm and hand function after stroke: A validity test of the hierarchical scoring system used in the Motor Assessment Scale for stroke, *Arch Phys Med Rehabil* 86:1609–1615, 2005.

Stokes EK, Neill O: Use of outcome measures in physiotherapy practice in Ireland from 1998 to 2003 and comparison to Canadian trends, *Physiother Can* 60:109–116, 2009.

Stokes EK, O'Neill D: The use of standardised assessments by physiotherapists, *British Journal of Therapy and Rehabilitation* 6:560–565, 1999.

Stroke Impact Scale: Online Available: www2.kumc.edu/coa/SIS/SIS_pg2.htm. Accessed July 22, 2009.

Van der Linden FAH, Kragt JJ, Klein M, et al: Psychometric evaluation of the multiple sclerosis impact scale (MSIS-29) for proxy use, *J Neurol Neurosurg Psychiatry* 76:1677–1681, 2005.

Van Hilten JJ, van der Zwan AD, Zwinderman AH, et al: Rating Impairment and Disability in Parkinson's disease: Evaluation of the Unified Parkinson's Disease Rating Scale, *Mov Disord* 9:84–88, 1994.

Verheyden G, Willems A, Ooms L, et al: Validity of the Trunk Impairment Scale as a measure of trunk performance in people with Parkinson's Disease, *Arch Phys Med Rehabil* 88:1304–1308, 2007.

Verheyden G, Hughes J, Jelsma J, et al: Assessing motor impairment of the trunk in patients with traumatic brain injury: reliability and validity of the Trunk Impairment Scale, *South African Journal of Physiotherapy* 62:23–28, 2006a.

Verheyden G, Nuyens G, Nieuwober A, et al: Reliability and validity of trunk assessment for people with multiple sclerosis, *Phys Ther* 86:66–76, 2006b.

Verheyden G, Nieuwboer A, Feys H, et al: Discriminant ability of the Trunk Impairment Scale: A comparison between stroke patients and healthy individuals, *Disabil Rehabil* 27:1023–1028, 2005.

Verheyden G, Nieuwboer A, Mertin J, et al: The Trunk Impairment Scale: a new tool to measure motor impairment of the trunk after stroke, *Clin Rehabil* 18:326–334, 2004.

Wang C, Hseuh I, Sheu C, et al: Psychometric properties of 2 simplified 3-level balance scales used for patients with stroke, *Phys Ther* 84:430–438, 2004.

Evaluating satisfaction

11

CHAPTER CONTENTS

Patient satisfaction: why measuring it is important

Understanding expectations and satisfaction with services has moved firmly into the healthcare domain and provides valuable additional information to clinical outcomes. It is becoming increasingly important in the provision of healthcare services. In the UK, all NHS trusts are required to survey a sample of their patients each year, and file a report to the Healthcare Commission (Coulter 2006). When evaluating a new model of service delivery, where clinical outcomes may not be significantly different, the perspective of the user of the service may be very informative in terms of how the service develops, e.g. a review of the introduction of an extended scope physiotherapy service in an emergency department demonstrated superior patient satisfaction with similar clinical outcomes (McClellan et al 2006). A positive experience may enhance the compliance with interventions, attendance at a service and can impact of overall health outcomes (Guldvog 1999)

While the surveys reviewed in Tables 11.1 and 11.2 may seem straightforward, the evaluation of user satisfaction is complex. Satisfaction depends on expectations which in turn can be influenced by knowledge and previous experience. Roush and Sonstroem (2001) interpret the findings of their development study in the light of Hertzberg's description of motivation of workers (Hertzberg 1968). They report four components to their satisfaction model: 'enhancer's, 'detractors', 'cost' and 'location'. They suggest that the 'enhancers' and 'detractors' are conceptually parallel to the 'satisfiers' and 'dissatisfiers' described by Hertzberg. The presence of 'satisfiers' does not automatically result in no dissatisfaction and vice versa. A patient may report satisfaction if his/her expectation is that the therapist will have a genuine interest in him/her and the therapist demonstrates that interest – this is considered an enhancer – a patient may be considered dissatisfied if the experience leaves the patient feeling that the therapist should have listened more carefully to what he/she was being told by the patient. Beattie et al (2002, 2005a,b) note that the patient–therapist interaction is reported to be a positive one if the patient feels that he or she was treated with respect, that questions were answered and that interventions were explained. In addition, having the same therapist for the course of treatment is also associated with satisfaction. Dissatisfaction occurs when there is a mismatch between expectations and experience. Kotler et al (2005) describe a number of reasons why there may be a mismatch between what a customer expects and what they experience and this mismatch is termed the 'quality gap'. The gap may occur for the following reasons:

- The service providers may not correctly perceive what the service user wants.
- The service provider may understand what the service user requires but may not clearly articulate the service standards to other staff to support the provision of the service to users.
- The service standards may be articulated but the staff is not supported, e.g. trained sufficiently, provided with sufficient resources, etc. to provide the appropriate service delivery.
- The external communications about the services, which will influence the service user's expectations, does not match the subsequent experience of the service user.
- There is a gap between the perceived service and the expected service.

The instruments reviewed in this chapter consider the patient/client's experience with physiotherapy services only; other more generic instruments are available for use in evaluating services, e.g. the SERVQUAL model (Youssef et al 1995, Curry & Sinclair 2002).

As described in Chapter 3, the checklist reported by Greenhalgh et al (1998) is the basis for the information provided in the tables that accompany this chapter on each outcome measure. Where relationships between variables are described in the context of validity and realiability, the statistical tests employed are co-efficients such as Pearson Product Moment and Spearman's Rank correlation co-efficient unless otherwise stated. Where details of the exact intra-class correlation (ICC) were provided in the primary source, it is included in the table and if not, the abbreviation ICC is used.

Table 11.1 Patient Satisfaction Questionnaire (PSQ)

Description	Perspective: Models informing development	Language	Availability & publications	User-centredness	Utility
13/14 closed questions scored on a 5-point scale with anchors of 'excellent' and 'bad/poor'.	Survey instruments should match the service provided. No physiotherapy (PT) instrument existed when this was developed. Review of various satisfaction survey instruments, particularly those focusing on single visits and available in French. No model articulated in support of the instrument.	French, German	Available – both French & German versions in Scascighini et al (2008) See Appendix 5 Monnin & Perneger (2002)	This survey instrument seeks to identify who referred the patient to the service, e.g. self-referral or other options. In addition, it explores the interactions with the PT and more operational issues such as the procedure for admission and the location.	The original French language version was developed for use in PT in a large teaching hospital – both inpatients and outpatients. The German version was tested on patients with orthopaedic problems, some of whom had surgery. They had experience of being inpatient and outpatients.

Validity			Reliability	
Face/content	Criterion including concurrent, predictive and diagnostic	Construct including convergent and discriminant	Relative	Internal consistency
French version Content validity: – initial survey was generated from a review of the literature and tested on a sample of 528 in- and outpatients (52% response rate to the postal survey). Principal component factor analysis yielded 3 factors accounting for 60% total variance. Item reduction was informed by a need to maintain content validity, internal consistency and to remove items that had a high number of missing values. This resulted in a final 14 items (from 25) and this new version was compared with the first iteration. *German version:* – translation and transcultural adaptation involved internationally recognized translation procedure. Tested on 123 outpatients 4 weeks after last PT appointment. Face validity of the items was established by professional consensus.		*French version* Construct: validity – Strong correlations between past experience and future intention and also between open and closed questions. Demographic characteristics not strongly related to scores. *German version* Construct: validity – strong correlations (Spearman rank) between the item scores and overall scores and between item identified as 'global assessment' and subscores.	*German version* Test–re-test ($n = 23$): Reported using Bland & Altman measures of agreement and ICC = 0.74–0.92	*French version* Cronbach's alpha = 0.77–0.90 *German version:* Cronbach's alpha = 0.94–0.95

Table 11.2 Physical Therapy Outpatient Satisfaction Survey (PTOPS) and European version (EPTOPS)

Description	Perspective: Models informing development	Language	Availability & publications	User-centredness	Utility
A 34-item instrument – statements scored with 5-point Likert scales: 1, strongly disagree; 2, disagree; 3, uncertain; 4, agree; 5, strongly agree.	Authors believe that PT is not closely monitored due to lack of appropriate instruments, hence its development. In their post-hoc discussion, the authors suggest that their findings are supportive of Hertzberg's (1968) work on motivators of employees.	American English, European English (EPTOPS)	American English in Roush & Sonstroem (1999) See Appendix 5 Casserley-Feeney et al (2008)	The view of patients attending outpatient PT services – both hospital-based and private practices. 6–10 min to complete.	This survey instrument examines 4 domains termed enhancers (aspects that make the experience more positive), detractors (aspects that make the experience less satisfying) as well as the experience of the location and the cost. The latter domain may be redundant for patients who incur no cost to attend the PT service.

Validity

Face/content	Construct including convergent and discriminant
American English version Face and content validity: a three-stage process was employed to establish the items for inclusion in the final instrument, the three samples included: 177, 257 and 173 outpatients from 21 facilities. The first iteration contained items reported frequently in the healthcare literature. Principal component factor and confirmatory factor analysis were performed on subsequent iterations, yielding a final version of 34 items, with 4 domains. *European English version* – translation and transcultural adaptation involved 3 Irish PTs and 3 PTs in the USA. Forward and backward translations were utilized to achieve linguistic equivalence.	*American English version* Construct validity: three subsamples were involved in the evaluation. Sample 1 examined the relationships between the PTOPS and a scale that measures social desirability. The Balanced Inventory of Desirable Responding has two subscales, impression management (IM) and self-deceptive enhancement (SDE) and explores the extent to which responses on the PTOPS actually capture the patient's experience rather than socially desirably responses. For the most part there was no such relationship indicating the PTOPS is free of the influence of social desirability. Discriminant validity: The PTOPTs was able to discriminate between patients reporting a particularly positive or particularly negative experience and between patients identified as 'high attendance' and 'low attendance'.

Reliability

Internal consistency
American English version Cronbach's alpha = 0.71–0.85

Table 11.3 MedRisk, MRPS

Description	Perspective: Models informing development	Language	Availability & publications	User-centredness	Utility
A 20-item instrument – 18 items and 2 global measures.	The authors note that two existing instruments developed for patients' satisfaction in PT present varied results, cost being influential in one sample and not in another and issues of importance varying between the two studies. They note that the purpose of their study was to develop an instrument closely associated with the overall satisfaction of patients.	American English, Spanish	Available in Beattie et al (2007) See Appendix 5 Beattie et al (2002, 2005a,b)	The view of patients attending outpatients for musculoskeletal conditions. Based on discussions with PTs and patients and the authors own views, items reflecting the personal aspects of the PT as well as system/ external aspects were included in the first iteration of the instrument.	Significant ongoing work is being completed on the ecological validity of the MedRisk Instrument.

Validity

Face/content

English version
Face validity: the initial 25-item instrument was evaluated by 2 experienced PTs producing an 18-item instrument for pilot testing; 191 patients completed the instrument and 4 global items. Regression analysis of a 20-item instrument accounted for 76% of the causes of patient satisfaction.
Content validity: 1868 patients (20% response rate) completed the 20-item instrument. Item reduction occurred after principal component factor analysis and oblimin rotation and yielded 2 versions of the instrument – a 2-component solution (10 items) and a 3-component solution (12 items).
Spanish version
Validation of the Spanish version was carried out on the original 20-item version. Forward and backward translation until consensus was achieved between the 4 translators; 250 instruments were completed.
Content validity:
Once again, principal component factor analysis revealed two factors accounting for 62% if the variance. Varimax rotation resulted in 7 items loading on a factor termed 'internal'; 3 items on a factor termed 'external', i.e. a 10-item instrument identical to the English language version.

Criterion including concurrent, predictive and diagnostic

English version
Concurrent validity: the scores on both the 10-item and 12-item versions compared strongly with 'overall satisfaction' and intention to return', with the 10-item versions having higher correlations (mean r = 0.756).
Discriminant validity: In a further larger sample of patients (n = 1449) the 10-item version and 2 global items were completed to explore if the instrument could differentiate between items related to interactions with the therapist 'internal' factor and 'external' factor. Confirmatory factor analysis supports the 2-factor hypothesis.
Concurrent validity
The scores on the 7 items relating to internal factor demonstrated strong correlations with 'overall' satisfaction (r = 0.82) and future intentions (r = 0.72). These scores were also significantly correlated for items making up the external factor.

Reliability

Absolute

English version
Standard error of the measurement (SEM) was used to evaluate reliability – the lower the SEM, the less error there was associated with the instrument; it was shown to be small in both studies: 0.2 for 10-item version, 0.24 for external factor and 0.19 for internal factor. Spanish version SEM = 0.16.

Internal consistency

English version
Cronbach's alpha for the 10-item version = 0.90 and for the 12-item version = 0.85. Cronbach's alpha for internal factor =0.90 and external factor = 0.87. Spanish version Cronbach's alpha = 0.90.

Table 11.4 Patient Satisfaction with Physical Therapy (PSPT)

Description	Perspective: Models informing development	Language	Availability & publications	User-centredness	Utility
7 general questions and 18 statements, which are scored with the 5-point Likert scale, where: 1 indicates strong disagreement with the statement and 5 indicates strong agreement.	Measuring patient satisfaction is important and attention has not been focused on PT. This instrument was developed to evaluate the satisfaction of patients with PT services. The authors used 5 previously reported domains of patient satisfaction to guide the development of the items in the instrument. The authors also used publications of the American Physical Therapy Association and other instruments found in the literature.	American English	Available in Goldstein et al (2000) See Appendix 5	7 questions asking about how the patient heard of the facility, previous experience, nature of PT problem as well as 18 questions of experience with the service. 6–10 min to complete	Only one publication on this instrument to date. Unclear how widely used it is.

Face/content	Validity		Reliability
	Criterion including concurrent, predictive and diagnostic	Construct including convergent and discriminant	Internal consistency
289 surveys were completed by outpatients at 12 practice settings. Content validity: the authors inferred this was good, as the included items were drawn from instruments used by PTs.	Construct validity: a multitrait-multimethod matrix examines the relationships (correlation coefficients) between all items in the instrument. The nature of the relationships supports the hypothesis that the instrument has multiple domains with appropriate levels of association between and within the domains. In addition, principal component factor analysis yielded one factor which accounted for 83% of the variance in the instrument.	Concurrent validity: 3 items were removed to become a criterion measure of 'best overall satisfaction'. A high degree of association was reported between scores on the criterion variables and the summary score of the remaining items.	Cronbach's alpha = 0.99

Table 11.5 Cystic Fibrosis Chest PT Satisfaction Survey

Description	Perspective: Models informing development	Language	Availability & publications	User-centredness	Utility
17 closed questions scored on a 5-point scale scored with 5-point Likert scale, where: 1 indicates strong disagreement with the statement and 5 indicates strong agreement.	Chest PT is an important part of the management of people with cystic fibrosis (CF). People with CF must use various airways clearance techniques (ACTs) and the survey was designed to enable research into patient satisfaction with various ACTs.	American English	See Appendix 5 Oermann et al (2000)	17 questions on chest PT and 3 general questions on overall satisfaction were devised by the authors which are designed to capture information on the patient's, or in the case of infants or young children, the care provider's views of perceived efficacy, convenience and comfort of (ACTs).	Only one publication on this instrument but may be useful in services for people with CF.

Validity			Reliability
Face/content	Criterion including concurrent, predictive and diagnostic	Construct including convergent and discriminant	Internal consistency
129 participants (response rate 39%) Criterion validity: in the absence of a *gold standard*, convergent validity was evaluated by comparing scores on the CPT Satisfaction with a measure of disease severity.	129 participants (response rate 39%) Construct validity: examined using confirmatory factor analysis, the authors hypothesized that there would be 4 factors: efficacy, convenience, comfort and overall satisfaction with the ACTs.	Test-re-test reliability: a sample of 16 (response rate 80%) repeated the survey instrument on two occasions (time between not reported). Reliability coefficients varied: 0.29 for convenience, 0.55 for comfort, 0.81 for efficacy.	Cronbach's alpha = 0.74–0.89

Table 11.6 Patient Satisfaction Questionnaire (PSQ)

Description	Perspective: Models informing development	Language	Availability & publications	User-centredness	Utility
A 38-item scale which has 6 domains: expectations, therapist, communication, organization, clinical outcome satisfaction. It is scored on a 5-point Likert scale, where: 1 indicates strong disagreement with the statement and 5 indicates strong agreement. The instrument contains both negative and positive statements, hence scoring is reversed for negative items.	The authors comment that scales developed in the USA that contain items relating to cost and access should be used in the UK with caution. Additional limitations in some extant scales are that patients were not involved in item generation and outcome was not considered. Hills & Kitchen (2007a,b) develop a model for patient satisfaction in the context of physiotherapy prior to the development of the satisfaction scale.	English (UK)	Presented in Hills & Kitchen (2007d) See Appendix 5 Hills & Kitchen (2007a,b,c,d)	The perspective of patients with both acute and chronic musculoskeletal problems attending as outpatients for physiotherapy.	Developed with services in the UK in mind; well described model to inform it development.

Validity		Reliability
Face/Content		Internal Consistancy
Face and content validity: a model is developed by the authors prior to 4 focus groups of patients with acute and chronic musculoskeletal conditions being conducted to explore issues relating to satisfaction. The results of the focus groups were used to inform the development of the instrument. Content validity: The initial 44-item instrument was completed by 120 patients and item reduction occurred following factor analysis.		Cronbach's alpha ≥ 0.8

References

Beattie PF, Pinto MB, Nelson MK, et al: Patient satisfaction with outpatient physical therapy: instrument validation, *Phys Ther* 82(6):557–564, 2002.

Beattie P, Turner C, Dowda M, et al: The MedRisk instrument for measuring patient satisfaction with physical therapy care: a psychometric analysis, *J Orthop Sports Phys Ther* 35 (1):24–32, 2005a.

Beattie P, Dowda M, Turner C, et al: Longitudinal continuity of care is associated with high patient satisfaction with physical therapy, *Phys Ther* 85(10):1046–1052, 2005b.

Beattie PF, Nelson RM, Lis A: Spanish language version of the Medrisk instrument for measuring patient satisfaction with physical therapy care (MRPS): Preliminary validation, *Phys Ther* 87(6):793–800, 2007.

Casserley-Feeney SN, Phelan M, Duffy F, et al: Patient satisfaction with private physiotherapy for musculoskeletal pain, *BMC Musculoskelet Disord* 9:50, 2008.

Coulter A: Can patients assess the quality of health care? *BMJ* 1;333(7557):1–2, 2006.

Curry A, Sinclair E: Assessing the quality of physiotherapy services using Servqual, *International Journal of Healthcare Quality Assurance* 15 (5):197–205, 2002.

Goldstein MS, Elliott SD, Guccione AA: The development of an instrument to measure satisfaction with physical therapy, *Phys Ther* 80(9):853–863, 2000.

Greenhalgh J, Long AF, Brettle AJ, et al: Reviewing and selecting outcome measures for use in routine practice, *J Eval Clin Pract* 4(4):339–350, 1998.

Guldvog B: Can patient satisfaction improve health among patients with angina pectoris? *Int J Qual Health Care* 11(3):233–240, 1999.

Hertzberg F: One more time: how do you motivate employees? *Harv Bus Rev* January/February:53–62, 1968.

Hills R, Kitchen S: Development of a model of patient satisfaction, *Physiother Theory Pract* 23 (5):255–271, 2007a.

Hills R, Kitchen S: Toward a theory of patient satisfaction with physiotherapy: exploring the concept of satisfaction, *Physiother Theory Pract* 23(5):243–254, 2007b.

Hills R, Kitchen S: Satisfaction with outpatient physiotherapy: focus groups to explore the views of patients with acute and chronic musculoskeletal conditions, *Physiother Theory Pract* 23(1):1–20, 2007c.

Hills R, Kitchen S: Satisfaction with outpatient physiotherapy: comparing the views if patients with acute and chronic musculoskeletal conditions, *Physiother Theory Pract* 23(1):21–36, 2007d.

Kotler P, Wong V, Saunders J, et al: *Principles of marketing*, ed 3, London, 2005, Prentice Hall.

McClellan CM, Greenwood R, Benger JR: Effect of an extended scope physiotherapy service on patient satisfaction and the outcome of soft tissue injuries an adult emergency department, *Emerg Med J* 23:384–387, 2006.

Monnin D, Perneger TV: Scale to measure patient satisfaction with physical therapy, *Phys Ther* 82 (7):682–691, 2002.

Oermann CM, Swank PR, Sockrider MM: Validation of an Instrument Measuring Patient Satisfaction with Chest Physiotherapy Techniques in Cystic Fibrosis, *Chest* 118(1):92–97, 2000.

Roush SE, Sonstroem RJ: Development of the Physical Therapy Outpatient Satisfaction Survey (PTOPS), *Phys Ther* 79(2):159–170, 1999.

Roush SE, Sonstroem RJ: Letters and responses, *Phys Ther* 81 (4):1061–1063, 2001.

Scascighini L, Angst F, Uebelhart D, et al: Translation, transcultural adaptation, reliability and validity of the Patient Satisfaction Questionnaire, in German, *Physiotherapy* 92:43–55, 2008.

Youssef F, Nel D, Bovaird T: Service quality in NHS hospitals, *J Manag Med* 9(1):66–74, 1995.

Appendix 1: Mobility

Introduction

This Appendix contains the outcome measures discussed in Chapter 7. In Tables 7.1 and 7.2 (in Ch. 7) there are listed links to a website where an electronic copy of the outcome variable is available.

This Appendix contains the following outcome measures:

- Emory Functional Ambulation Profile (E-FAP) Scale and Modified Emory Functional Ambulation Profile Scale (mE-FAP)
- Hierarchic Assessment of Balance and Mobility (HABAM)
- Elderly Mobility Scale and Modified Elderly Mobility Scale
- Rivermead Mobility Index and Modified Rivermead Mobility Index
- University of Alabama at Birmingham Study of Aging Life Space Assessment
- High Level Mobility Assessment Tool (HiMAT)
- The Activities-Specific Balance Confidence (ABC) Scale
- Physiotherapy Functional Mobility Profile
- Trinity Test of Mobility.

© 2011, Elsevier Ltd.
DOI: 10.1016/B978-0-443-06915-4.00012-7

Emory Functional Ambulation Profile Scale and Modified Emory Functional Ambulation Profile Scale

The inclusion of manual assistance is the modification to the original version of the E-FAP.

The E-FAP is composed of five subtasks: (1) Floor, (2) Carpet, (3) Up and Go, (4) Obstacles and (5) Stairs. Each subject is given a rest period between performances of the subtasks, long enough for the researcher to explain and demonstrate the next component. Each subject post-stroke is instructed to use an assistive device or receive manual assistance as needed and to wear a gait belt during performance of all subtasks. The researcher designated as primary researcher demonstrates, provides instructions, and answers the subject's questions. The primary researcher and secondary researcher each record performance times for all five subtasks on separate data collection forms. Upon completion of the entire data collection session, each researcher calculates a total E-FAP score.

Introduction

The primary researcher provides an explanatory overview of the five subtasks comprising the E-FAP. Prior to performance of each subtask, the primary researcher explains and demonstrates the subtask. The subject is informed that the performance of each subtask is timed and is instructed to ask clarification questions at any time.

Floor

Set-up: A 1-m strip of masking tape is placed on the hard-surfaced floor at the starting point. Five meters ahead of the starting point, a 2-cm piece of masking tape marks the end-point. A small piece of tape is used to mark the end-point so that subjects do not decelerate in anticipation of the finish line.

1. The primary researcher explains while demonstrating the 'Floor' subtask: 'When I say "go", walk at your normal, comfortable pace until I say "stop".'
2. The primary researcher assists the subject as needed in placing toes on starting line tape.
3. The primary researcher says 'go' and the primary and secondary researchers simultaneously press stopwatches to begin timing.
4. The subject walks towards the primary researcher, who is standing 1 m beyond the end-point of the 5-m distance. The secondary researcher walks alongside the subject as the subject traverses the 5-m distance.
5. The primary and secondary researchers simultaneously press stopwatches to stop as the subject's lead foot crosses the end-point. The primary researcher tells the subject to 'stop' when he or she is beyond the end-point.
6. The primary and secondary researchers record times on separate data collection forms.

Carpet

Set-up: A piece of short pile carpet, no less than 7 m long and 2 m wide, is taped securely to the floor. The starting point is marked with a 1-m strip of masking tape. The end-point is marked exactly 5 m from the starting point with a 2-cm piece of masking tape. Both the starting point and end-point are at least 1 m from the edge of the carpet.

1. The primary researcher explains while demonstrating the Carpet subtask: 'When I say "go", walk at your normal, comfortable pace until I say "stop".'
2. The primary researcher assists the subject as needed in placing toes on starting line tape.
3. The primary researcher says 'go' and the primary and secondary researchers simultaneously press stopwatches to begin timing.
4. The subject walks towards the primary researcher who is standing 1 m beyond the end-point of the 5-m distance. The secondary researcher walks alongside the subject as the subject traverses the 5-m distance.
5. The primary and secondary researchers simultaneously press stopwatches to stop timing as the subject's lead foot crosses the end-point. The primary researcher tells the subject to 'stop' when he or she is beyond the end-point.
6. The primary and secondary researchers record times on separate data collection forms.

Up and Go

Set-up: A standard armchair with a 46-cm seat height is placed on the hard-surfaced floor. Three meters away, a 1-m strip of black tape is placed on the floor.

1. The primary researcher explains while demonstrating the Up and Go subtask: 'Next, you will sit in this chair with your back against the back of the chair and your arms resting on the armrests. When I say "go" you will stand up from the chair, walk at your normal comfortable pace past this line where I will be standing, turn around, walk back to the chair, and sit down, making sure your back is against the back of the chair.'

2. The subject assumes a sitting position in the chair. The primary researcher stands at the 3-m point marked with masking tape. The secondary researcher stands beside the chair and prepares to walk with the subject.

3. The primary researcher says 'go' and primary and secondary researchers simultaneously press stopwatches to begin timing.

4. The primary researcher monitors the line to ensure both of subject's feet cross the line before turning around.

5. The primary and secondary researchers stop timing when the subject is fully seated with back against the chair.

6. The primary and secondary researchers record times on separate data collection forms.

Obstacles

Set-up: A 1-m piece of masking tape is placed on a hard-surfaced floor to mark the starting point. A brick is placed on the floor at the 1.5-m mark and the 3-m mark. A 40-gallon rubber rubbish bin is placed at the 5-m mark.

1. The primary researcher explains while demonstrating the Obstacles subtask: 'When I say "go" walk forwards at your normal, comfortable pace and step over each brick. Then, walk around the rubbish bin from either the left or right. Then walk back stepping over the bricks again. Continue walking until I say "stop".'

2. The primary researcher assists the subject as needed in placing toes on the starting line.

3. The primary researcher says 'go' and the primary and secondary researchers simultaneously press stopwatches to begin timing.

4. When the subject begins walking, the primary researcher steps back 1 m beyond the end line, while the secondary researcher walks with the subject.

5. When the subject's foot crosses the end line, the primary and secondary researchers

simultaneously press stop on their stopwatches. The researcher tells the subject to 'stop' when he or she is beyond the end line, while the secondary researcher simultaneously presses the stopwatches to stop timing. The primary researcher tells the subjects to 'stop' when he or she is beyond the end line.

6. The primary and secondary researchers record times on separate data collection forms.

Stairs

Set-up: Stairs with four steps, hand railings, and the following measurements are utilized: 26.04-cm stair depth, 75.57-cm stair width, 15.24-cm stair height, 76.20-cm platform depth, and 75.57-cm platform width. A 1-m piece of masking tape is placed 25 cm from the base of the first step.

1. The primary researcher explains while demonstrating the Stairs subtask: 'When I say "go" walk up the stairs at your normal, comfortable pace to the top of the stairs, turn around, and come back down. You may use the handrails if needed. I will follow behind you for safety.'

2. The primary researcher assists the subject as needed in placing toes on starting tape.

3. The primary researcher says 'go' and primary and secondary researchers simultaneously press stopwatches to begin timing.

4. The primary researcher follows the subject up the stairs to guard.

5. The primary and secondary researchers press stopwatches to stop timing when subject's non-lead foot comes into firm contact with the floor.

6. The primary and secondary researchers record times on separate data collection forms.

Scoring the Emory Functional Ambulation Profile

1. Researchers multiply the time recorded for each subtask by the appropriate factor according to the level of assistive device used during that subtask.

2. Researchers record the product in the cell corresponding to the appropriate subtask and level of assistive device.

3. Researchers repeat this procedure for each column/subtask.

4. Researchers sum the five subtask scores to obtain the E-FAP total score.

5. All total scores are computed without the factor for assistance device, for the purposes of statistical testing.

Hierarchic assessment of balance and mobility (HABAM)

	Score	1	2	3	4	5	6	7	8	9	10
						Day					
Balance											
Stable ambulation	21										
Stable dynamic standing	14										
Stable static standing	10										
Stable dynamic sitting	7										
Stable static sitting	5										
Impaired static sitting	0										
Transfers											
Independent	18										
1 person standby	12										
1 person minimal assist	11										
1 person assist	7										
2 person assist	3										
Total lift	0										
Mobility											
Unlimited	26										
Limited >50m	25										
Unlimited with aid	21										
With aid >50 m	18										
With aid 8–50m	15										
1 person standby ± aid	12										
1 person hands-on ± aid	9										
Lying-sitting independently	7										
Positions self in bed	4										
Needs positioning in bed	0										

Reproduced from Rockwood K, Rockwood MRH, Andrew MK, Mitnitski A. Reliability of the Hierarchical Assessment of Balance and Mobility in Frail Older Adults. Journal of the American Geriatrics Society 2008 56:1213-1217 with permission of Wiley-Blackwell Publishing.

Elderly Mobility Scale and Modified Elderly Mobility Scale

Elderly Mobility Scale

Scoring key

Lying to sitting

2 Independent
1 Supervision or help of 1 person
0 Help of ≥2 people
(maximum score 2)

Sitting to lying

2 Independent
1 Supervision or help of 1 person
0 Help of ≥2 persons
(maximum score 2)

Sitting to standing

3 Independent in under 3 s
2 Independent in over 3 s
1 Supervision or help of 1 person (verbal or physical)
0 Help of ≥2 persons
(maximum score 3)

Stand

3 Stands without support* and able to reach
2 Stands without support* but needs support to reach
1 Stands but needs support
0 Stands only with physical help (help of another person)

*Support means the need of the upper limbs to steady self
(maximum score 3)

Gait

3 Independent including (the use of sticks)
2 Independent with walking frame
1 Mobile with walking aid but erratic/unsafe turning (needs occasional supervision)
0 Needs physical help to walk or constant supervision
(maximum score 3)

Timed walk (6 m)

3 under 15 s
2 16–30 s
1 Over 30 s
0 Unable to cover 6 m
(maximum score 3)

Functional reach

4 Over 16 cm
2 8–16 cm
0 Under 8 cm or unable
(maximum score 4)
Total maximum score possible 20.

Reproduced from Smith R 1994 Validation and Reliability of the Elderly Mobility Scale. Physiotherapy 80(11): 744-747 with permission from Elsevier.

Modified Elderly Mobility Scale

Scoring key

Lying to sitting

2 Independent
1 Supervision or help of 1 person
0 Help of 2 or more people

(maximum score 2)

Sitting to lying

2 Independent
1 Supervision or help of 1 person
0 Help of 2 or more persons

(maximum score 2)

Sitting to standing

3 Independent in 3 s or less
2 Independent in more than 3 s
1 Supervision or help of 1 person (verbal or physical)
0 Help of 2 or more persons

(maximum score 3)

Standing balance

3 Stands without support* and can lift arms forward and out to the sides
2 Stand without support* but requires support to lift arms
1 Stands with support*
0 Stands with physical help (help of another person)

*Support means the need of the upper limbs to balance
(maximum score 3)

Gait

3 Independent including the use of stick or elbow crutch (unilateral support)
2 Independent with walking frame or 2 sticks/crutches (bilateral support)
1 Walks with or without walking aid but erratic/unsafe turning (requires occasional supervision)
0 Requires physical help to walk or constant supervision

(maximum score 3)

Timed walk (6 m)

3 15 s or less
2 16–30 s
1 Over 30 s
0 Unable to cover 6 m

(maximum score 3)

Functional reach

4 Over 20 cm
2 10–20 cm
0 Under 10 cm/unable

(maximum score 4)
Total maximum score possible 20

Guidelines

Lying to sitting, sitting to lying

The patient is instructed to transfer from supine lying to sitting on the edge of the bed with or without his/her feet on the ground and then return to supine lying. Assistive devices such as monkey pole and raised backrest are not permitted.

2 The patient can transfer independently without verbal or physical assistance
1 The patient requires supervision, verbal or physical assistance of 1 person
0 The patient requires assistance of 2 or more persons.

Sitting to standing

Using a chair with armrests and with a height of 48 cm. The patient is instructed to rise from sitting to standing with or without using the armrests. Timing commences when the patient starts the task (e.g. when the patient starts to move his/her feet back, leans forward, etc.) and stops when the patient stands upright with or without support as required.

3 The patient can rise independently from sitting to standing in 3 s or less
2 The patient can rise independently in more than 3 s
1 The patient requires the use of assistive devices, verbal or physical assistance of 1 person in order to rise from sitting to standing
0 The patient requires the assistance of 2 or persons.

Standing balance

In the standing position, with support if required, the patient is instructed to lift his/her arms forward and then sideways to a level of 90 degrees.

3   The patient can stand upright without support and lift his/her arms forward and sideways as if to reach for something within arms length (i.e. NOT stretching)

2   The patient can stand without support but requires to steady himself/herself on walking aid or furniture when attempting to reach

1   The patient can stand independently by steadying himself/herself on a walking aid or furniture

0   The patient requires physical assistance of one or more persons (i.e. is not safe or unable to stand unaided).

Gait

The patient is instructed to walk, with his/her normal walking aid, a distance that is comfortable for the patient, to turn, change direction, stop, and start and to open and shut a door (e.g. toilet door).

3   The patient walks independently without a walking aid alternatively with a stick/elbow crutch (i.e. unilateral support). The patient can walk safely, is able to turn, to change direction, stop and start without help or supervision

2   The patient can walk safely with a walking frame, rollator, 2 crutches or 2 sticks (i.e. bilateral support). The patient can turn, change direction, stop and start without supervision

1   The patient walks with or without a walking aid however requires occasional supervision, e.g. when turning, changing direction, opening or shutting a door, etc.

0   The patient requires physical assistance to walk or constant supervision.

Timed walk

Walking speed is timed over a distance of 6 m. The patient starts walking approximately 1 m before the therapist starts timing. The patient walks at their normal walking speed with walking aid if required.

3   The patient covers the distance in 15 s or less

2   The patient covers the distance in 16–30 s

1   The patient covers the distance in more than 30 s

0   The patient is unable to cover the distance or unable to walk.

Modified functional reach

1. The physiotherapist explains and demonstrates how to carry out the task. A trial run is carried out followed by an attempt that is measured. If the patient misunderstands the instructions or the task is not fully carried out the test is re-done.

2. The patient stands with his/her right or left side against a wall. A measuring tape is attached to the wall at the height of the patient's acromion.

3. The patient is instructed to make a fist with his/her hand against the wall and to lift the arm to shoulder height (90 degrees flexion) without reaching forward.

4. The position of the third metacarpal joint is noted against the measuring tape.

5. The patient is then instructed to: 'Reach as far forward as you can without moving your feet. You may not touch the wall with your fist or arm.' The patient should maintain their fist in the outstretched position. The patient may flex the trunk and hips.

6. In the outstretched position, the position of the third metacarpophalangeal joint will once again be in the outstretched position the position of the third metacarpophalangeal joint will once again be noted as in point 4.

7. The patient must be able to return to the starting position without assistance, touching the wall or moving his/her feet for the test to be valid.

8. Functional reach is the distance between the third metacarpophalangeal joint at the start position and the outstretched position.

   4   The patient can reach over 20 cm

   2   The patient can reach between 10 and 20 cm

   0   The patient is unable to reach 10 cm or cannot stand without support.

Reproduced from Linder A, Winkvist L, Nilsson L, Sernet N. Evaluation of the Swedish Version of the Modified Elderly Mobility Scale (Swe M-EMS) in patients with acute stroke. Clinical Rehabilitation 2005 20:584-597, with permission from Sage Publications.

Rivermead Mobility Index and Modified Rivermead Mobility Index

Rivermead Mobility Index

Instructions

The patient is asked the following 15 questions, and observed (for item 5). A score of 1 is given for each 'yes' answer. Note that most require independence from personal help, but method is otherwise unimportant.

Q		A Question	Comment
1	Turning over in bed	Do you turn over from your back to your side without help?	
2	Lying to sitting	From lying in bed, do you get up to sit on the edge of the bed on your own?	
3	Sitting balance	Do you sit on the edge of the bed without holding on for 10 seconds?	
4	Sitting to standing	Do you stand up from any chair in less than 15 seconds and stand there for 15 seconds (using hand and with an aid if necessary)?	
5	Standing unsupported	Observe standing for 10 seconds without any aid or support.	
6	Transfer	Do you manage to move, e.g. from bed to chair without any aid or support?	
7	Walking inside, with an aid if needed	Do you walk 10 metres, with an aid or furniture if necessary, but with no standby help?	
8	Stairs	Do you manage a flight of stairs without help?	
9	Walking outside (even ground)	Do you walk around outside, on pavements without help?	
10	Walking inside, with no aid	Do you walk 10 metres inside with no calliper, splint, aid, or use of furniture, and no standby help?	
11	Picking off floor	If you drop something on the floor, do you manage to walk 5 metres to pick it up and then walk back?	
12	Walking outside (uneven ground)	Do you walk over uneven ground, e.g. grass, gravel, dirt, snow, ice?	
13	Bathing	Do you get in/out of bath or shower unsupervised and wash self?	
14	Up and down four steps	Do you manage to go up and down 4 steps with no rail and no help (can use aid if necessary)?	
15	Running	Do you run 10 metres without limping in 4 seconds (fast walk acceptable)?	

Modified Rivermead Mobility Index

Patient's name: _____

Assessor's name: _____

Test date: _____

Test location: _____

Scoring:

0 unable to perform
1 assistance of 2 people
2 assistance of 1 person
3 requires supervision or verbal instruction
4 requires and aid or an appliance
5 independent

Item	Score
1	Turning over Please turn over from your back to your side
2	Lying to sitting Please sit up on the side of the bed
3	Sitting balance Please sit on the edge of the bed (the assessor times the patient for 10 s)
4	Sitting to standing Please stand up from your chair (the patient takes less than 15 s
5	Standing Please remain standing
6	Transfers Please go from your bed to the chair and back again
7	Walking indoors Please walk for 10 metres in your usual way
8	Stairs Please climb up and down this flight of stairs in your usual way

University of Alabama at Birmingham Study of Aging Life Space Assessment

Name: _____

Date: _____

These questions refer to your activities within the past month:

Life-space level	Frequency	Independence	Score
During the past 4 weeks, have you been to ...	How often did you get there?	Did you use aids or equipment? Did you need help from another person?	Level (*x*) Frequency (*x*) Independence (*x*)
Level 1			
Other rooms of your home besides where you sleep? Yes **1** No **0**	<1/ week **1** 1–3 times/ week **2** 4–6 times/ week **3** Daily **4**	1 = Personal assistance 1.5 = Equipment only 2 = No equipment or personal assistance	
		Level 1 score:	
Level 2			
An area outside your home such as your porch, deck or patio, hallway or garage, in your own yard or driveway? Yes **1** No **0**	<1/ week **1** 1–3 times/ week **2** 4–6 times/ week **3** Daily **4**	1 = Personal assistance 1.5 = Equipment only 2 = No equipment or personal assistance	
		Level 2 score:	
Level 3			
Places in your neighbourhood, other than your own yard or apartment building? Yes **1** No **0**	<1/ week **1** 1–3 times/ week **2** 4–6 times/ week **3** Daily **4**	1 = Personal assistance 1.5 = Equipment only 2 = No equipment or personal assistance	
		Level 3 score:	
Level 4			
Places outside your neighbourhood but within your town Yes **1** No **0**	<1/ week **1** 1–3 times/ week **2** 4–6 times/ week **3** Daily **4**	1 = Personal assistance 1.5 = Equipment only 2 = No equipment or personal assistance	
		Level 4 score:	

Continued

Life-space level							Independence	Score
			Frequency					
Level 5								
Places outside your town?	Yes	No	<1/ week	1–3 times/ week	4–6 times/ week	Daily	1 = Personal assistance 1.5 = Equipment only 2 = No equipment or personal assistance	
	1	0	1	2	3	4		
							Level 5 score:	
Total score:							Sum of levels 1–5	

High Level Mobility Assessment Tool (HiMAT)

Date: _____

Date of accident: _____

Diagnosis: _____

Affected side left/right: _____

PATIENT
IDENTIFICATION
LABEL

Item				Score				
	Performance	0	1	2	3	4	5	
Walk	Seconds		>6.6	5.4–6.6	5.4–6.6	<4.3	X	
Walk backward	Seconds		>13.3	8.1–13.3	5.8–8.0	<5.8	X	
Walk on toes	Seconds		>8.9	7.0–8.9	5.4–6.9	<5.4	X	
Walk over obstacle	Seconds		>7.1	5.4–7.1	4.5–5.3	<4.5	X	
Run	Seconds		>2.7	2.0–2.7	1.7–1.9	<1.7	X	
Skip	Seconds		>4.0	3.5–4.0	3.0–3.4	<3.0	X	
Hop forward (more-affected leg)	Seconds		>7.0	5.3–7.0	4.1–5.2	<4.1	X	
Bound (more-affected leg)	1 cm 2 3		<80	80–103	104–132	>132	X	
Bound (less-affected leg)	1 cm 2 3		<82	82–105	106–129	>129	X	
Upstairs dependent (rail *or* not reciprocal. If not, score 5 and rate below)			<22.8	14.6–22.8	12.3–4.5	<12.3	X	
Upstairs independent (no rail *or* not reciprocal. If not, score 0 and rate above)			>9.1	7.6–9.1	6.8–7.5	<6.8	X	
Downstairs dependent (rail *or* not reciprocal. If not, score 5 and rate below)			>24.3	17.6–24.3	12.8–17.5	<12.8	X	
Downstairs independent (no rail *and* reciprocal. If not, score 0 and rate above)			>8.4	6.6–8.4	5.8–6.5	<5.8	X	

Total HiMAT score = 54.

Instructions

Subject suitability: The HiMAT is appropriate for assessing people with high-level balance and mobility problems. The minimal mobility requirement for testing is independent walking over 20 m without gait aids. Orthoses are permitted.

Item testing

Testing takes 5–10 min. Patients are allowed one practice trial for each item.

Instructions

Patients are instructed to perform at their maximum safe speed except for the bounding and stair items.

- Walking: The middle 10 m of a 20 m trial is timed.
- Walk backward: As for walking.
- Walk on toes: As for walking. Any heel contact during the middle 10 m is recorded as a fail.
- Walk over obstacle: As for walking. A house brick is placed across the walkway at the mid-point. Patients must step over the brick without contacting it. A fail is recorded if patients step around the brick or make contact with the brick.
- Run: The middle 10 m of a 20 m trial is timed. A fail is recorded if patients fail to have a consistent flight phase during the trial.
- Skipping: The middle 10 m of a 20 m trial is timed. A fail is recorded if patients fail to have a consistent flight phase during the trial.
- Hop forward: Patients stand on their more affected leg and hop forward. The time to hop 10 m is recorded.
- Bound (affected): A bound is a jump from one leg to the other with a flight phase. Patients stand behind a line on their less affected leg, hands on hips, and jump forward landing on their more affected leg. Each bound is measured from the line to the heel of the landing leg. The average of three trials is recorded.

- Bound (less-affected): Patients stand behind a line on their more affected leg, hands on hips, and jump forward landing on their less affected leg. The average of three trials is recorded.
- Up stairs: Patients are asked to walk up a flight of 14 stairs as they normally would and at their normal speed. The trial is recorded from when the patient starts until both feet are at the top. Patients who use a rail or a non-reciprocal pattern are scored on Up Stairs Dependent. Patients who ascend the stairs reciprocally without a rail are scored on Up Stairs Independent and get an additional 5 points in the last column of Up Stairs Dependent.
- Down stairs: As for Up stairs.

Scoring

All times and distances are recorded in the 'performance' column. The corresponding score for each item is then circled and each column is then sub-totalled. Subtotals are then added to calculate the HiMAT score.

Reproduced from Williams G P, Robertson V, Greenwood K M, Goldie P A, Morris M E. The high-level mobility assessment tool (HiMAT) for traumatic brain injury Part 2: Content validity and discriminability. Brain Injury 2004 19(10): 833-843, with permission from Informa Healthcare

The Activities-specific Balance Confidence (ABC) Scale

Instructions to participants

For each of the following, please indicate your level of confidence in doing the activity without losing your balance or becoming unsteady from choosing one of the percentage points on the scale form 0% to 100%. If you do not currently do the activity in question, try and imagine how confident you would be if you had to do the activity. If you normally use a walking aid to do the activity or hold onto someone, rate your confidence as if you were using these supports. If you have any questions about answering any of these items, please ask the administrator.

Scoring

For each of the following activities, please indicate your level of self-confidence by choosing a corresponding number from the following rating scale:

0%	10	20	30	40	50	60	70	80	90	100%
No confidence					$\longrightarrow$					Completely confident

How confident are you that you will not lose your balance or become unsteady when you . . .

1. Walk around the house? ___%

2. Walk up or down stairs? ___%

3. Bend over and pick up a slipper from the front of a cupboard floor ___%

4. Reach for a small can off a shelf at eye level? ___%

5. Stand on your tiptoes and reach for something above your head? ___%

6. Stand on a chair and reach for something? ___%

7. Sweep the floor? ___%

8. Walk outside the house to a car parked in the driveway? ___%

9. Get into or out of a car? ___%

10. Walk across a parking lot to the shopping centre? ___%

11. Walk up or down a ramp? ___%

12. Walk in a crowded shopping centre where people rapidly walk past you? ___%

13. Are bumped into by people as you walk through the shopping centre? ___%

14. Step onto or off an escalator while you are holding onto a railing? ___%

15. Step onto or off an escalator while holding onto parcels such that you cannot hold onto the railing? ___%

16. Walk outside on icy pavements? ___%

Reproduced from Powell, LE & Myers AM. The Activities-specific Balance Confidence (ABC) Scale. *J Gerontol Med Sci* 1995; 50(1): M28-34, with permission from Oxford University Press

Physiotherapy Functional Mobility Profile

	7 Independent	6 Slow/ Device	5 Supervision cueing/set-up	4 Minimum assistance client 99–75%	3 Moderate assistance client 74–50%	2 Maximum assistance client 49–25%	1 Total assistance client 24–0%	Score
Bed mobility Rolling Bridging		e.g. bedrail						
Lie to sit At side of bed								
Sit to stand	From any height chair							
Sitting balance Feet supported Side of bed	Protective reflexes normal	Tolerates external displacement	Self-displacement outside base	Self-displacement within base	Maintains balance with no displacement			
Standing balance Double stance		External displacement	Self-displacement outside base	Self-displacement within base	Maintains balance with no displacement			
Transfers Bed, chair, wheelchair. Toilet			Supervised	Minimum assistance	Pivot with 1 assistant	Pivot with 2 assistants	Life (2–3 person) or mechanical lift	
Wheelchair locomotion Indoors, manual or electric		50 m in 5 min turns, door, sits 3% grade	15 m independent: or needs cueing for 50 m	15 m with supervision	15 m with occasional assistant	15 m with constant assistance	Less than 15 m	
Ambulation Indoors	50 m turns 180° backward 3 steps		50 m with supervision or 15 m independent	50 m with 1 person steadying	50 m with 1 assistant	Min 15 m with 1 assistant	2 assistants or cannot walk 15 m	
Stairs 12–14 indoors up and down		e.g. hand rail	Supervision for 12 steps or 6 independent	12 with minimum assistance	12 with 1 assistant	4 with assistant	2 assistants or is carried	
Total score								

Reproduced from Platt W, Bell B, Kozak J. Physiotherapy Functional Mobility Profile: A Tool for Measuring Functional Outcome in Chronic Care Clients. Physiotherapy Canada 1998: 47-74, with permission from University of Toronto Press. © Canadian Physiotherapy Association 2009.

Trinity Test of Mobility

Bed rise (0–6)

Ability to rise from lying on a plinth, bring legs over the edge of the bed and sit up. In the case of patients with stroke or orthopaedic conditions, use the side of the plinth that will optimise performance and repeat assessments consistently on this side. The patient should use the number of pillows normally used when sleeping.

Instruction: I'd like you to get up from lying and sit over the edge of the bed, as quickly as you can.

0 Requires hoist/mechanical aid
1 Requires assistance of 2
2 Requires assistance of 1 for the leg(s) and/or trunk and/or arms
3 Requires verbal cueing/prompting to complete task or because of safety issues
4 Uses compensatory strategies. Below are some examples of compensatory strategies that may be employed, the list is not meant to be definitive:
   • Pulls off bed rails/monkey pole
   • Takes a long duration or demonstrates *repeated use* of upper extremities to push off bed
   • Discontinuity of trunk elevation and leg motion off bed
   • LE use: multiple motions, poor clearance of heels, pulls with leg to aid motion
   • Hands grasp thigh or buttocks to aid trunk movement
   • Rolls onto one side and uses contralateral upper extremity (UE) for push-off
5 Independent, no compensatory strategies, transient use of upper extremities is acceptable
6 Independent in 3 s or less.

Start this section by asking the patient to see if they are able to stand up from the chair without using their arms. If they can, then ask them to repeat the activity using the instructions below.

Sit to stand (0–6)

Ability to stand from a chair that allows the patient to sit with their knees and hips at approximately 90 degrees and their feet flat on the floor. The patient may use one or both upper extremities, if necessary, but only after trying without using the upper extremities first.

Instruction: 'I'd like you to get up out of the chair and stand up straight, as quickly as you can. I'd like you to try this without using your hands.'

0 Requires mechanical aid
1 Requires assistance of 2
2 Requires assistance of 1
3 Requires verbal cueing for safety and/or task description – supervision
4 Uses compensatory strategies; some examples are listed below – you may wish to add others
   • Use of UEs
   • Repeated forward flexion of trunk to initiate the movement, i.e. use of momentum
   • Cushions on chair enable independence by reducing the height from which the patient has to rise
   • _____
   • _____
5 Independent in >2 s
6 Independent in 2 s or less.

Standing ability and stability (0–13)

The ability to stand in the most upright posture for a given patient. With the therapist sitting/standing in front of the patient, ask the patient to stand up. One arm may be supported to allow the patient to position their feet, if the patient needs help positioning their feet; the therapist carries this out. The patient is asked if they are ready, support is removed and timing is begun (relevant for 3 onwards). The patient's arms should remain close the body.

0 Unable to stand unsupported
1 Able to stand with assistance of 1
2 Able to stand with assistance of an aid
3 Immediate standing with no physical support
4 Feet apart, with broad base (>20 cm between medial aspect heels) – eyes open (EO) – maintains for 10 s
5 Feet apart, with broad base (>20 cm between medial aspect heels) – eyes closed (EC) – maintains for 10 s
6 Feet apart, with normal base – EO – maintains for 10 s
7 Feet apart, with normal base – EC – maintains for 10 s

8   Feet together – EO – maintains for 10 s

9   Feet together – EC – maintains for 10 s

10 Semi-tandem, the heel of one foot is placed beside the base of the first toe of the opposite foot – EO – maintains for 10 s

11 Semi-tandem, the heel of one foot is placed beside the base of the first toe of the opposite foot – EC – maintains for 10 s

12 Tandem, the heel of one foot is placed in front of the toes of the other foot – EO – maintains for 10 s

13 Tandem, the heel of one foot is placed in front of the toes of the other foot – EC – maintains for 10 s

Reach and lift (0–6)

The patient is asked to lift a textbook or equipment catalogue from a standard gym table, hand it to the physiotherapist who places his/her receiving hand at a height that requires the patients to achieve 90 degrees flexion at the shoulder or in the case of limited shoulder movement, the greatest range available. In the case of one non-functioning upper extremity, one arm may be used.

This is a timed task. It commences with the patient standing.

Instructions: 'When I say "go", I want you to take the book from the table and hand it to me.'

0 Unable

1 Able with assistance of 1, for the purposes of stability

2 Requires use of compensatory strategies

Needs to hold object, e.g. aid or table, on reaching up

3 Independent in >6 s

4 Independent in 4.6–6 s

5 Independent in 2.6–4.5 s

6 Independent in ≤2.5 s.

Bend and Reach (0–6)

Place a cone on the floor approximately 1 metre away from the patient on their dominant or unaffected side in the case of upper extremity dysfunction. Ask them to pick it up from the floor and stand up.

This is a timed task. The patient is standing to start the test.

Instruction: 'When I say "go", I want you to pick the cone up from the floor.'

0 Unable

1 Able with assistance of 1, for the purposes of stability, throughout task

2 Requires use of compensatory strategies
   - Needs to lean on object to lean down or come up
   - Inadequate knee flexion – reaches from trunk
   - Needs assistance on rising

3 Independent in >6 s

4 Independent in 4.6–6 s

5 Independent in 2.6–4.5 s

6 Independent in ≤2.5 s

Repeated sit to stand (0–8)

You will know already if the patient can go from sit to stand without arms, from the earlier test. The patient is asked to stand up and sit down five times, from a standard chair.

Time starts at the initial sitting position to the final standing position at the fifth stand.

Instruction: 'When I say "go", I want you to stand up and sit down as quickly as you can, five times. Please try not to use your arms to help you push up.'

Verbal cueing to count the number of stands is allowed. No encouragement should be given.

0 Unable to complete

1 Completed in ≥16.7 s, with UE use

2 Completed in 13.7–16.6 s, with UE use

3 Completed in 11.2–13.6 s, with UE use

4 Completed in a time ≤11.1 s, with UE use

5 Completed in ≥16.7 s, without UE use

6 Completed in 13.7–16.6 s, without UE use

7 Completed in 11.2–13.6 s, without UE use

8 Completed in a time ≤11.1 s, without UE use

Gait ability (0–12)

This test assesses gait ability and speed, at the higher levels of performance. The patient is asked to walk 'at your normal comfortable speed' along a stretch marked out on the floor in the gym or with cones, if necessary. Approximately 2 m acceleration and deceleration are allowed. The patient uses their assistive device. A frame includes a rollator or motorized frame or two crutches. A cane also incorporates the use of one crutch or one elbow crutch.

Timing occurs over 10 m of the course, following the length of acceleration.

0 Unable to mobilize or complete 10 m

1 Requires assistance of 2 to mobilize

2 Requires maximum assistance

3 Requires moderate assistance

4 Requires contact guard assistance/verbal cueing/supervision

5   Completes with frame independently in >30 s

6   Completes independently with a frame in <30 s

7   Completes independently with a cane in >10 s (male)/>11 s (female)

8   Completes independently with a cane in 7–10 s (male)/7–11 s (female)

9   Completes independently with a cane in <7 s (male)/<7.5 s (female)

10 Completes independently with no aid >10 s (male)/>11 s (female)

11 Completes independently with no aid in 7–10 s (male)/7–11 s (female)

12 Completes independently with no aid in <7 s (male)/<7.5 s (female)

Appendix 2: Physical activity

Introduction

This Appendix contains the outcome measures discussed in Chapter 8. In Tables 8.1 and 8.2 (in Ch. 8) there are details about how to purchase the activity monitors and a link to the PASE and PAR-7 website, hence this section contains the one remaining measure of physical activity: the Physical Activity Disability Survey (PADS).

© 2011, Elsevier Ltd.
DOI: 10.1016/B978-0-443-06915-4.00013-9

The Physical Activity Disability Survey (PADS)

This questionnaire asks you questions about the types of exercise and physical activities you participated in over the last week and the time you spent doing these activities.

If you compared the activities you took part in over the last week to the activities you would take part in on a typical week, would you say you did (please circle):

Much less than usual	Less than usual	About the same as usual	More than usual	Much more than usual
1	2	3	4	5

1. Exercise

Did you exercise in the last week? Exercise is any activity you do on a regular basis for the primary purpose of increasing or maintaining fitness. Please note: this does not include activities you do for leisure or recreation.

Yes ☐   No ☐

If No, please go to Question 2
If Yes, what kind of exercise did you do?
Please list the exercise activities below that you did in the last week for the primary purpose of maintaining or improving your health and fitness. For each activity indicate the activity type and intensity (using the keys below), how many days per week you did the activity and how many minutes per day.

Activity types

A = Aerobic Exercise (aerobic activities are those exercises done for a sustained period of time which result in an increase in your heart rate and breathing rate, e.g. walking, jogging, attending an aerobics class, cycling, etc.)

S = Strength Exercise (strength activities, e.g. lifting weights or using elastic bands or weight training machines, pilates, core body strengthening and stability, tai chi, etc.)

F = Flexibility Exercise (flexibility refers to activities that involve muscle stretching, e.g. yoga, etc.)

Intensity

L = Light activities (don't sweat or breathe heavily)

M = Moderate activities (breathe a little harder and may sweat)

V = Vigorous activities (breathe hard and sweat)

Activity type (A, S or F)	Activity	Days/ Week	Minutes/ Day	Intensity (L, M or V)

Exercise Matrix

	Light	Moderate	Vigorous
Flexibility	1	2	4
Strength	2	4	8
Aerobic	3	6	12

Activity Score (for each activity listed) = Days/week × Minutes/day × Exercise Matrix Score

Total Exercise Score = sum of all Activity Scores:

$SCORE\ 1 = ln(Total\ Exercise\ Score/60) + 0.1)$

2. Leisure time physical activity

Did you participate in any sports, recreational, or leisure time activities in the last week? These activities may not necessarily result in sustained increases in heart rate and breathing rate. Examples include hiking, boating, skiing, dancing, bowling and sports activities.

Yes ☐	No ☐

If No, please go to Question 3
If Yes, what type of activities did you do?
Please list the leisure time physical activities below that you did in the last week for leisure or recreation. For each activity indicate the activity type and intensity (using the keys below), how many days per week you did the activity and how many minutes per day. Do not list activities here that you have already listed previously in this questionnaire.

Activity types

    E = Endurance (endurance activities are leisure time physical activities that you maintain for a sustained period of time that make you sweat and breathe a little harder than usual, e.g. tramping/hiking, tennis, dancing, skiing, sports fishing, sexual activity, etc.)

  NE = Non-endurance (non-endurance activities are leisure time physical activities that you might do in shorter bouts of activity and/or do not cause you to sweat and breathe a

little harder, e.g. boating, fishing by the jetty, bowling, etc.)

Intensity

    L = Light activities (don't sweat or breathe heavily)
  M = Moderate activities (breathe a little harder and may sweat)
  V = Vigorous activities (breathe hard and sweat)

Activity type (E or NE)	Activity	Days/ Week	Minutes/ Day	Intensity (L, M or V)

Leisure Time Physical Activity (LTPA) Matrix

	Light	Moderate	Vigorous
Non-endurance	1	2	4
Endurance	2	4	8

Activity Score (for each activity listed) = Days/week × Minutes/day × LTPA Matrix Score

Total LTPA Score = sum of all Activity Scores

SCORE 2 = ln(Total LTPA Score/60) + 0.1)

3. General activity

3.1. From Monday to Friday last week, how many waking hours a day did you spend inside your home (please tick one)?

<6 h a day	☐
6–8 h a day	☐
9–10 h a day	☐
11–12 h a day	☐
≥13 h a day	☐

Scores

- <6 h a day = 4
- 6–8 h a day = 3
- 9–10 h a day = 2
- 11–12 h a day = 1
- ≥13 h a day = 0

3.2. On Saturday and Sunday last week, how many waking hours a day did you spend inside your home (please tick one)?

<6 h a day	☐
6–8 h a day	☐
9–10 h a day	☐
11–12 h a day	☐
≥13 h a day	☐

Scores

- <6 h a day = 4
- 6–8 h a day = 3
- 9–10 h a day = 2
- 11–12 h a day = 1
- ≥13 h a day = 0

SCORE 3 = (3.1 + 3.2)/2

3.3. During the last week, how many hours a day did you sleep including naps?

☐	Hours

3.4. During the last week, how many hours a day were you sitting or lying down (including work), but excluding sleeping?

☐	Hours

SCORE 4 = 24 − (3.3 + 3.4)

3.5. During the last week did you do any indoor household activities, such as cleaning, food preparation, childcare activities, etc?

Yes	☐	No	☐

If No, please go to Question 3.6

If Yes, please list all the indoor activities that required some physical activity (e.g. cleaning, hanging washing, food preparation, etc.) that you did in the last week. Please also include here any physical activities you did as a part of your role as caregiver (e.g. parenting activities). For each activity, indicate how many days per week you did the activity and how many minutes per day. Do not list activities here that you have already listed previously in this questionnaire.

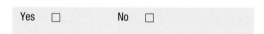

Activity	Days/Week	Minutes/Day

Activity Score (for each activity listed) = Days/week × Minutes/day

Indoor Activity Score = sum of all Activity Scores

SCORE 5 = ln(Indoor Activity Score/60) + 0.1)

3.6. During the last week did you do any outdoor household activities, such as gardening, walking to and from shops, etc?

Yes	☐	No	☐

If No, please go to Question 3.7

If Yes, please list all the outdoor activities that required some physical activity (e.g. gardening, mowing lawns, walking to shops) that you did in the last week. For each activity indicate how many days per week you did the activity and how many minutes per day. Do not list activities here that you have already listed previously in this questionnaire.

Activity	Days/Week	Minutes/Day

Activity Score (for each activity listed) = Days/week × Minutes/day

Outdoor Activity Score = sum of all Activity Scores

$$SCORE\,6 = ln(Outdoor\,Activity\,Score/60) + 0.1)$$

3.7. During the last week did you climb any stairs at home?

Yes ☐   No ☐

If No, please go to Question 3.8

3.7a. If YES, how many flights of stairs do you have at home (one flight of stairs is 5–10 steps)?

☐   Flights

3.7b. If YES, how many times a day did you climb these stairs in the last week?

☐   Times a day

Total Flights = 3.7a × 3.7b

SCORE 7:
- No flights = 0
- 1–6 flights/day = 1
- 7–10 flights/day = 2
- ≥11 flights/day = 3

3.8. How much assistance do you need to perform the activities of daily living, such as dressing and bathing (please tick one)?

Without assistance	☐
Some assistance	☐
Full assistance	☐

SCORE 8:
- Without assistance = 2
- Some assistance = 1
- Full assistance = 0

4. Therapy

During the last week did you receive physiotherapy or occupational therapy or another type of therapy that involves physical activity? If you have already listed therapy-related activities previously in this questionnaire, DO NOT complete this section.

Yes ☐   No ☐

If No, please go to Question 5
How many days a week did you receive a therapy that involved physical activity in the last week?

☐   Days/week

How long did each activity-based therapy session last?

	Minutes
☐	

SCORE 9:
- No therapy = 0
- 1 session/week = 1
- ≥2 sessions/week = 2

5. Employment/school

Are you currently employed, participate in any volunteer work or do you attend school?

Employed/Attend school/Volunteer work	☐
Not employed/Do not attend school/ Do not do any volunteer work	☐
Retired	☐

If you are NOT EMPLOYED, DO NOT ATTEND SCHOOL, DO NOT DO ANY VOLUNTEER WORK or ARE RETIRED, please go to Question 6

5.1. For most of your work/school day, do you:

Move around	☐
Stand	☐
Sit	☐

SCORE 10:
- Move around = 2
- Stand = 1
- Sit = 0
- Not employed = 0

5.2. During the last week did you climb any stairs while at work/school?

Yes ☐	No ☐

If No, please go to Question 5.3

5.2a. If Yes, how many flights of stairs do you have at work/school (one flight of stairs is 5–10 steps)?

	Flights
☐	

5.2b. If Yes, how many times a day did you climb these stairs in the last week?

	Times a day
☐	

Total Flights = 5.2a × 5.2b

SCORE 11:
- Not employed = 0
- No flights = 0
- 1–6 flights/day = 1
- 7–10 flights/day = 2
- ≥11 flights/day = 3

5.3. During the last week did you get any physical activity in your transportation to and from work/school (e.g. walking to work)?

Yes ☐	No ☐

If No, please go to Question 6
If Yes, please list all the transportation physical activity you did in the last week (e.g. walking or wheeling a wheelchair to and from work). For each activity indicate how many days per week you did the activity and how many minutes per day. Do not list activities here

that you have already listed previously in this questionnaire.

Activity	Days/Week	Minutes/Day

Activity Score (for each activity listed) = Days/week × Minutes/day

Transport Activity score = sum of all Activity Scores

SCORE 12:

- Not employed = 0
- No transport activity = 0
- 1 to 60 min/week = 1
- $\geq$61 min/week = 2

6. Wheelchair users

During the last week did you use a wheelchair?

Yes ☐   No ☐

If No, stop this questionnaire.
If Yes, during the time that you were awake, how much time a day did you spend in your wheelchair in the last week (please tick one)?

All day	☐
Most of the day	☐
A few hours	☐

What type of wheelchair did you primarily use in the last week (please tick one)?

Manual	☐
Power	☐

If POWER WHEELCHAIR, stop this questionnaire. If MANUAL, did you push your own wheelchair at any time during the last week?

Yes ☐   No ☐

If No, stop this questionnaire.
If Yes, on average, how many minutes a day did you push yourself in your wheelchair in the last week?

<60 min	☐
$\geq$60 min	☐

SCORE 13:

- No wheelchair use = 0
- Pushed for <60 min = 1
- Pushed for $\geq$60 min = 2

Scoring subscales

Exercise/Leisure time physical activity

$$(SCORE\ A) = (0.7071((SCORE\ 1 - 0.535)/2.344)) + (0.7071((SCORE\ 2 + 1.571)/1.643))$$

General

$$(SCORE\ B) = (0.3748(SCORE\ 3 - 2.031)/1.338) + (0.4481(SCORE\ 4 - 8.350)/4.977) + (0.4399(SCORE\ 5 - 1.314)/1.962) + (0.3811(SCORE\ 6 + 0.490)/1.742) + (0.3045(SCORE\ 7 - 0.914)/1.108) + (0.4766(SCORE\ 8 - 1.704)/0.585)$$

Therapy

$$(SCORE\ C) = SCORE\ 9$$

Employment

$$(SCORE\ D) = (0.6021(SCORE\ 10 - 0.301)/0.704) + (0.6290(SCORE\ 11 - 0.351)/0.783) + (0.4918(SCORE\ 12 - 0.099)/0.374)$$

Wheelchair

$$(SCORE\ E) = SCORE\ 13$$

Total score

$$TOTAL\ PADS = (0.5349(SCORE\ A/1.074)) + (0.6369(SCORE\ B/1.540)) + (-0.0967(SCORE\ C - 0.104)/0.378) + (0.5005(SCORE\ D/1.184)) + (-0.2198(SCORE\ E - 0.165)/0.497)$$

Reproduced from Kayes N M, Schluter P J, McPherson K M, Taylor D, Kolt G S. Clinical Rehabilitation 23:534-543, 2009 © Reprinted by permission of Sage Publications.

Appendix 3: Fatigue

Introduction

This Appendix contains the outcome measures discussed in Chapter 10. In Tables 10.1 and 10.2 (in Ch. 10) there are listed links to a website where an electronic copy of the outcome variable is available.

This Appendix contains the following outcome measures:

- Fatigue Severity Scale, Fatigue Severity Scale for use in Multiple Sclerosis
- Fatigue Impact Scale and Modified Fatigue Impact Scale
- Barrow Neurological Institute (BNI) Fatigue Scale
- Brief Fatigue Inventory
- Modified Piper Fatigue Scale
- Multidimensional Fatigue Inventory.

DOI: 10.1016/B978-0-443-06915-4.00014-0

Fatigue Severity Scale

9-Item Scale: Fatigue Severity Scale (FSS)

1. My motivation is lower when I am fatigued
2. Exercise brings on my fatigue
3. I am easily fatigued
4. Fatigue interferes with my physical functioning
5. Fatigue causes frequent problems for me
6. My fatigue prevents sustained physical functioning
7. Fatigue interferes with carrying out certain duties
8. Fatigue is among my three most disabling symptoms
9. Fatigue interferes with my work, family or social life.

Patients are instructed to choose a number from 1 to 7 that indicates their degree of agreement with each statement, where 1 indicates *strongly disagree* and 7 indicates *strongly agree*.

5-Item Fatigue Severity Scale for patients with multiple sclerosis

Patients are instructed to choose a number from 1 to 7 that indicates their degree of agreement with each statement where 1 indicates *strongly disagree* and 7 indicates *strongly agree*.

1. My fatigue interferes with responsibilities
2. My fatigue interferes with work
3. My fatigue interferes with physical activity
4. My fatigue causes frequent problems
5. I am easily fatigued.

Reproduced from Mills RJ, Young CA, Nicholas RS, Pallant JF, Tennant A. Rasch analysis of the Fatigue Severity Scale in multiple sclerosis. 2009 Multiple Sclerosis 15:81-87, with permission from Sage Publications.

Fatigue Impact Scales

Please read each statement carefully and place an 'X' in the box that indicates best:
How much of a problem fatigue has been for you today.
Please check *one* box for each statement and do not skip any items.

	No problem (0)	Small problem (1)	Moderate problem (2)	Big problem (3)	Extreme problem (4)
Cognitive dimension					
Because of my fatigue:					
I feel less alert					
I have difficulty paying attention for a long period					
I feel like I cannot think clearly					
I find that I am more forgetful					
I find it difficult to make decisions					
I am less motivated to do anything that requires thinking					
I am less able to finish tasks that require thinking					
I find it difficult to organize my thoughts when I am doing things at home or at work					
I feel slowed down in my thinking					
I find it hard to concentrate					
Physical dimension					
Because of my fatigue:					
I am more clumsy					
I have to be careful about pacing my physical activities					
I am less motivated to do anything that requires physical efforts					
I have trouble maintaining physical effort for long periods					
My muscles feel much weaker than they should					
My physical discomfort is increased					
I am less able to complete tasks that require physical effort					
I worry about how I look to other people					
I have to limit my physical activities					
I require more frequent or longer periods of rest					

Continued

	No problem (0)	Small problem (1)	Moderate problem (2)	Big problem (3)	Extreme problem (4)
Psychosocial dimension					
Because of my fatigue:					
I feel that I am more isolated from social contacts					
I have to reduce my workload or responsibilities					
I am more moody					
I work less effectively (this applies to work inside or outside the home)					
I have to rely more on others to help me or to do things for me					
I have difficulty planning activities ahead of time					
I am more irritable and more easily angered					
I am less motivated to engage in social activities					
My ability to travel outside home is limited					
I have few social contacts outside my own home					
Normal day-to-day events are stressful for me					
I avoid situations that are stressful for me					
I have difficulty dealing with anything new					
I feel unable to meet demands that people place on me					
I am less able to provide financial support for my self and my family					
I engage in less sexual activity					
I am less able to deal with emotional issues					
I have difficulty participating in family activities					
I am not able to provide as much emotional support to my family as I should					
Minor difficulties seem like major difficulties					

Barrow Neurological Institute (BNI) Fatigue Scale

Please rate the extent to which each of the items below has been a problem for you since your injury. You should chose only ONE number from 0–7 on the scale below when making your response.

Rarely a problem		Occasional problem but not frequent	A frequent problem		A problem most of the time	
0	1	2 3	4	5	6	7

1. How difficult is it for me to maintain my energy throughout the day? ☐
2. How difficult is it for me to participate in activities because of fatigue? ☐
3. How difficult is it for me to stay awake during the day? ☐
4. How difficult is it for me to complete a task without becoming tired? ☐
5. How difficult is it for me to stay alert during activities? ☐
6. How difficult is it for me to build my energy level once I wake up in the morning? ☐
7. How difficult is it for me to stay out of my bed during the day? ☐
8. How difficult is it for me to stay alert when I am not involved in something? ☐
9. How difficult is it for me to attend to something without becoming sleepy? ☐
10. How difficult is it for me to last the day without taking a nap? ☐
11. Please circle your OVERALL level of fatigue since your injury:

No problem										Severe problem
0	1	2	3	4	5	6	7	8	9	10

Reproduced from Borgaro S, Gierok S, Caples H, Kwasnica C. Fatigue after brain injury: initial reliability study of the BNI Fatigue Scale. Brain Injury 2004 18(7):685-690, with permission from Informa Healthcare.

Brief Fatigue Inventory (BFI)

Throughout our lives, most of us have times when we feel very tired or fatigued. Have you ever felt unusually tired or fatigued in the last week?

Yes ☐   No ☐

1. Please rate your fatigue (weariness, tiredness) by circling the one number that best describes your fatigue right NOW.

No fatigue										**As bad as you can imagine**
0	1	2	3	4	5	6	7	8	9	10

2. Please rate your fatigue (weariness, tiredness) by circling the one number that best describes your usual level of fatigue during past 24 hours.

No fatigue										**As bad as you can imagine**
0	1	2	3	4	5	6	7	8	9	10

3. Please rate your fatigue (weariness, tiredness) by circling the one number that best describes your WORST level of fatigue during past 24 hours.

No fatigue										**As bad as you can imagine**
0	1	2	3	4	5	6	7	8	9	10

4. Circle the one number that describes how, during the past 24 hours, fatigue has interfered with your:
A. General activity

Does not interfere										**Completely interferes**
0	1	2	3	4	5	6	7	8	9	10

B. Mood

Does not interfere										**Completely interferes**
0	1	2	3	4	5	6	7	8	9	10

C. Walking ability

Does not interfere										**Completely interferes**
0	1	2	3	4	5	6	7	8	9	10

D. Normal work (includes both work outside the home and daily chores)

Does not interfere   **Completely interferes**

0	1	2	3	4	5	6	7	8	9	10

E. Relations with other people

Does not interfere   **Completely interferes**

0	1	2	3	4	5	6	7	8	9	10

F. Enjoyment of life

Does not interfere   **Completely interferes**

0	1	2	3	4	5	6	7	8	9	10

This material is reproduced from Mendoza T, Wang X, Cleeland C, Morrissey M, Johnson B, Wendt J, Huber S 1999 The Rapid Assessment of Fatigue Severity in Cancer Patients. Cancer 1999 85:1186-1196 © American Cancer Society with the permission of Wiley-Liss, Inc., a subsidiary of John Wiley & Sons, Inc.

Modified Piper Fatigue Scale

Many individuals can experience a sense of unusual or excessive tiredness whenever they become ill, receive treatment, or recover from their illness/treatment. This unusual sense of tiredness is not usually relieved by either a good night's sleep or by rest. Some call this symptom 'fatigue' to distinguish it from the usual sense of tiredness.

For each of the following questions, please fill in the space provided with the response that best describes the fatigue you are experiencing now or for today. Please make every effort to answer each question to the best of your ability. If you are not experiencing fatigue now or for today, fill in the circle indicating '0' for your response.

1. How long have you been feeling fatigue? (Tick one response only).

1. Not feeling fatigue ☐

2. Minutes ☐

3. Hours ☐

4. Days ☐

5. Weeks ☐

6. Months ☐

7. Other (Please describe) _____

2. To what degree is the fatigue you are feeling now causing you distress?

None										A Great Deal
0	1	2	3	4	5	6	7	8	9	10

3. To what degree is the fatigue you are feeling now interfering with your ability to complete your work or school activities?

None										A Great Deal
0	1	2	3	4	5	6	7	8	9	10

4. To what degree is the fatigue you are feeling now interfering with your ability to socialize with your friends?

None										A Great Deal
0	1	2	3	4	5	6	7	8	9	10

5. To what degree is the fatigue you are feeling now interfering with your ability to engage in sexual activity?

None										A Great Deal
0	1	2	3	4	5	6	7	8	9	10

6. Overall, how much is the fatigue which you are now experiencing interfering with your ability to engage in the kind of activities you enjoy doing?

None **A Great Deal**

| 0 | 1 | 2 | 3 | 4 | 5 | 6 | 7 | 8 | 9 | 10 |

7. How would you describe the degree of intensity or severity of the fatigue which you are experiencing now?

Mild **Severe**

| 0 | 1 | 2 | 3 | 4 | 5 | 6 | 7 | 8 | 9 | 10 |

8. To what degree would you describe the fatigue which you are experiencing now as being?

Pleasant **Unpleasant**

| 0 | 1 | 2 | 3 | 4 | 5 | 6 | 7 | 8 | 9 | 10 |

9. To what degree would you describe the fatigue which you are experiencing now as being?

Agreeable **Disagreeable**

| 0 | 1 | 2 | 3 | 4 | 5 | 6 | 7 | 8 | 9 | 10 |

10. To what degree would you describe the fatigue which you are experiencing now as being?

Protective **Destructive**

| 0 | 1 | 2 | 3 | 4 | 5 | 6 | 7 | 8 | 9 | 10 |

11. To what degree would you describe the fatigue which you are experiencing now as being?

Positive **Negative**

| 0 | 1 | 2 | 3 | 4 | 5 | 6 | 7 | 8 | 9 | 10 |

12. To what degree would you describe the fatigue which you are experiencing now as being?

Normal **Abnormal**

| 0 | 1 | 2 | 3 | 4 | 5 | 6 | 7 | 8 | 9 | 10 |

13. To what degree are you now feeling:

Strong										Weak
0	1	2	3	4	5	6	7	8	9	10

14. To what degree are you now feeling:

Awake										Sleepy
0	1	2	3	4	5	6	7	8	9	10

15. To what degree are you now feeling:

Lively										Listless
0	1	2	3	4	5	6	7	8	9	10

16. To what degree are you now feeling:

Refreshed										Tired
0	1	2	3	4	5	6	7	8	9	10

17. To what degree are you now feeling:

Energetic										Unenergetic
0	1	2	3	4	5	6	7	8	9	10

18. To what degree are you now feeling:

Patient										Impatient
0	1	2	3	4	5	6	7	8	9	10

19. To what degree are you now feeling:

Relaxed										Unrelaxed
0	1	2	3	4	5	6	7	8	9	10

20. To what degree are you now feeling:

Exhilarated										Depressed
0	1	2	3	4	5	6	7	8	9	10

21. To what degree are you now feeling:

Able to concentrate										Unable to concentrate
0	1	2	3	4	5	6	7	8	9	10

22. To what degree are you now feeling:

Able to remember										Unable to remember
0	1	2	3	4	5	6	7	8	9	10

23. To what degree are you now feeling:

Able to think clearly										Unable to think clearly
0	1	2	3	4	5	6	7	8	9	10

24. Overall, what do you believe is *most* directly contributing to or causing your fatigue?

_____

_____

_____

25. Overall, the *best* thing you have found to relieve your fatigue is:

_____

_____

_____

26. Is there anything else you would like to add that would describe your fatigue better to us?

_____

_____

_____

27. Are you experiencing any other symptoms right now?

_____

_____

_____

Reproduced with permission from Piper BF, Dibble SL, Dodd MJ, Weiss MC, Slaughter RE, Paul SM The revised Piper Fatigue Scale: psychometric evaluation in women with breast cancer. Oncology Nursing Forum 1998 25(4):677-684

Multidimensional Fatigue Inventory (MFI-20)

By means of the following statements we would like to get an idea of how you have been feeling *lately*. There is, for example, the statement:

'I feel relaxed'

If you think that this is *entirely true*, that indeed you have been feeling relaxed lately, please, place an X in the extreme left box; like this:

Yes, that is true	X					No, that is not true

The more you *disagree* with the statement, the more you can place an X in the direction of 'No, that is not true'. Please, do not miss out a statement and place one X next to each statement.

1.	I feel fit	Yes, that is true					No, that is not true
2.	Physically I feel only able to do a little	Yes, that is true					No, that is not true
3.	I feel very active	Yes, that is true					No, that is not true
4.	I feel like doing all sorts of nice things	Yes, that is true					No, that is not true
5.	I feel tired	Yes, that is true					No, that is not true
6.	I think I do a lot in a day	Yes, that is true					No, that is not true
7.	When I am doing something, I can keep my thoughts on it	Yes, that is true					No, that is not true
8.	Physically I can take on a lot	Yes, that is true					No, that is not true
9.	I dread having to do things	Yes, that is true					No, that is not true
10.	I think I do very little in a day	Yes, that is true					No, that is not true
11.	I can concentrate well	Yes, that is true					No, that is not true
12.	I am rested	Yes, that is true					No, that is not true
13.	It takes a lot of effort to concentrate on things	Yes, that is true					No, that is not true
14.	Physically I feel I am in a bad condition	Yes, that is true					No, that is not true
15.	I have a lot of plans	Yes, that is true					No, that is not true
16.	I tire easily	Yes, that is true					No, that is not true
17.	I get little done	Yes, that is true					No, that is not true
18.	I don't feel like doing anything	Yes, that is true					No, that is not true
19.	My thoughts easily wander	Yes, that is true					No, that is not true
20.	Physically, I feel I am in an excellent condition	Yes, that is true					No, that is not true

From Smets E, Garsen B, Bonke B, De Haes J 1995 The Multidimensional Fatigue Inventory (MFI) Psychometric Qualities of an instrument to assess fatigue. Journal of Psychometric Research 39(5):315-325, reprinted with permission.

Appendix 4: Neurological rehabilitation

Introduction

This Appendix contains the outcome measures discussed in Chapter 10. In Tables 10.1 and 10.2 (in Ch. 10) there are listed links to a website where an electronic copy of the outcome variable is available.

This Appendix contains the following outcome measures:

- Trunk Impairment Scale

- Multiple Sclerosis Impact Scale Version 2
- New Freezing of Gait Questionnaire
- Postural Assessment Scale for Stroke – 5 and 3 level scoring versions
- Short Parkinson's Evaluation Scale (SPES/SCOPA)
- Motor Assessment Scale with alternative scoring for upper limb sections.

© 2011, Elsevier Ltd.
DOI: 10.1016/B978-0-443-06915-4.00015-2

Trunk Impairment Scale (TIS)

The starting position for each item is the same. The patient is sitting on the edge of a bed or treatment table without back and arm support. The thighs make full contact with the bed or table; the feet are hip width apart and placed flat on the floor. The knee angle is 90°. The arms rest on the legs. If hypertonia is present, the position of the hemiplegic arm is taken as the starting position. The head and trunk are in a midline position.

If the patient scores 0 on the first item, the total score for the TIS is 0.

Each item of the test can be performed three times. The highest score counts. No practice session is allowed. The patient can be corrected between the attempts.

The tests are verbally explained to the patient and can be demonstrated if needed.

Item		
Static sitting balance		
1. Starting position		
	Patient falls or cannot maintain starting position for 10 seconds without arm support	☐ 0
	Patient can maintain starting position for 10 seconds	☐ 2
Note	If score = 0, then TIS total score = 0	
2. Starting position		
Therapist crosses the unaffected leg over the hemiplegic leg	Patient falls or cannot maintain sitting position for 10 seconds without arm support	☐ 0
	Patient can maintain sitting position for 10 seconds	☐ 2
3. Starting position		
Patient crosses the unaffected leg over the hemiplegic leg	Patient falls	☐ 0
	Patient cannot cross the legs without arm support on bed or table	☐ 1
	Patient crosses the legs but displaces the trunk more than 10 cm backwards or assists crossing with the hand	☐ 2
	Patient crosses the legs without trunk displacement or assistance	☐ 3
Total static sitting balance		☐/7
Dynamic sitting balance		
1. Starting position		
Patient is instructed to touch the bed or table with hemiplegic elbow (by shortening the hemiplegic side and lengthening the unaffected side) and return to the starting position	Patient falls, needs support from an upper extremity or the elbow does not touch the bed or table	☐ 0
	Patient moves actively without help; elbow touches bed or table	☐ 1
Note	If score = 0, then item 3 scores 0	
2. Repeat item 1	Patient demonstrates no or opposite shortening/lengthening	☐ 0
	Patient demonstrates appropriate shortening/lengthening	☐ 1
Note	If score = 0, then item 3 scores 0	

3. Repeat item 1	Patient compensates. Possible compensations are: (1) use of upper extremity, (2) contralateral hip abduction, (3) hip flexion (if elbow touches bed or table further then proximal half of femur), (4) knee flexion, (5) sliding of the feet	☐ 0
	Patient moves without compensation	☐ 1
4. Starting position Patient is instructed to touch the bed or table with the unaffected elbow (by shortening the unaffected side and lengthening the hemiplegic side) and return to the starting position Note	Patient falls, needs support from an upper extremity or the elbow does not touch the bed or table	☐ 0
	Patient moves actively without help; elbow touches bed or table	☐ 1
	If score = 0, then items 5 and 6 score 0	
5. Repeat item 4	Patient demonstrates no or opposite shortening/lengthening	☐ 0
	Patient demonstrates appropriate shortening/lengthening	☐ 1
6. Repeat item 4	Patient compensates. Possible compensations are: (1) use of upper extremity, (2) contralateral hip abduction, (3) hip flexion (if elbow touches bed or table further than proximal half femur), (4) knee flexion, (5) sliding of the feet	☐ 0
	Patient moves without compensation	☐ 1
7. Starting position Patient is instructed to lift pelvis from bed or table at the hemiplegic side (by shortening the hemiplegic side and lengthening the unaffected side) and return to the starting position Note	Patient demonstrates no or opposite shortening/lengthening	☐ 0
	Patient demonstrates appropriate shortening/lengthening	☐ 1
	If score = 0, then item 8 scores 0	
8. Repeat Item 7	Patient compensates. Possible compensations are: (1) use of upper extremity, (2) pushing off with the ipsilateral foot (heel loses contact with the floor)	☐ 0
	Patient moves without compensation	☐ 1
9. Starting position Patient is instructed to lift pelvis from bed or table at the unaffected side (by shortening the unaffected side and lengthening the hemiplegic side) and return to the starting position	Patient demonstrates no or opposite shortening/lengthening	☐ 0
	Patient demonstrates appropriate shortening/lengthening	☐ 1
10. Repeat item 9	Patient compensates. Possible compensations are: (1) use of upper extremities, (2) pushing off with ipsilateral foot (heel loses contact with floor)	☐ 0
	Patient moves without compensation	☐ 1
Total dynamic sitting balance		☐/10

Continued

Coordination

1. Starting position

Patient is instructed to rotate upper trunk 6 times (every shoulder should be moved forward 3 times); first side that moves must be hemiplegic side, head should be fixated in starting position	Hemiplegic side is not moved three times	☐ 0
	Rotation is asymmetrical	☐ 1
	Rotation is symmetrical	☐ 2

2. Repeat item 1 within 6 seconds

	Rotation is asymmetrical	☐ 0
	Rotation is symmetrical	☐ 1

3. Starting position

Patient is instructed to rotate lower trunk 6 times (every knee should be moved forward 3 times), first side that moves must be hemiplegic side, upper trunk should be fixated in starting position	Hemiplegic side is not moved three times	☐ 0
	Rotation is asymmetrical	☐ 1
	Rotation is symmetrical	☐ 2
Note	If score = 0, then item 4 scores 0	

4. Repeat item 3 within 6 seconds

	Rotation is asymmetrical	☐ 0
	Rotation is symmetrical	☐ 1

Total coordination	☐/6

Total Trunk Impairment Scale	☐/23

Reproduced from Verheyden G, Neiuwboer A, Mertin J, Preger R, Keikens C, De Weerdt W. The Trunk Impairment Scale: a new tool to measure motor impairment of the truck after stroke. Clinical Rehabilitation 2004 18:326-334, with permission from Stage Publications.

Multiple Sclerosis Impact Scale (MSIS-29) Version 2

The following questions ask for your views about the impact of MS on your day-to-day life during the past 2 weeks.

For each statement, please circle the ONE number that best describes your situation.

Please answer all questions.

		Not at all	A little	Moderately	Extremely
In the past 2 weeks, how much has your MS limited your ability to:					
1.	Do physically demanding tasks?	1	2	3	4
2.	Grip things tightly (e.g. turning on taps)?	1	2	3	4
3.	Carry things?	1	2	3	4
In the past 2 weeks, how much have you been bothered by:					
4.	Problems with your balance?	1	2	3	4
5.	Difficulties moving about indoors?	1	2	3	4
6.	Being clumsy?	1	2	3	4
7.	Stiffness?	1	2	3	4
8.	Heavy arms and/or legs?	1	2	3	4
9.	Tremor of your arms or legs?	1	2	3	4
10.	Spasms in your limbs?	1	2	3	4
11.	Your body not doing what you want it to do?	1	2	3	4
12.	Having to depend on others to do things for you?	1	2	3	4
13.	Limitations in your social and leisure activities at home?	1	2	3	4
14.	Being stuck at home more than you would like to be?	1	2	3	4
15.	Difficulties using your hands in everyday tasks?	1	2	3	4
16.	Having to cut down the amount of time you spent on work or other daily activities?	1	2	3	4
17.	Problems using transport (e.g. car, bus, train, taxi, etc.)?	1	2	3	4
18.	Taking longer to do things?	1	2	3	4
19.	Difficulty doing things spontaneously (e.g. going out on the spur of the moment)?	1	2	3	4
20.	Needing to go to the toilet urgently?	1	2	3	4
21.	Feeling unwell?	1	2	3	4
22.	Problems sleeping?	1	2	3	4
23.	Feeling mentally fatigued?	1	2	3	4
24.	Worries related to your MS?	1	2	3	4
25.	Feeling anxious or tense?	1	2	3	4

Continued

		Not at all	A little	Moderately	Extremely
26.	Feeling irritable, impatient, or short tempered?	1	2	3	4
27.	Problems concentrating?	1	2	3	4
28	Lack of confidence?	1	2	3	4
29.	Feeling depressed?	1	2	3	4

Reprinted with the permission of the author, Dr. Jeremy Hobart.

New Freezing of Gait Questionnaire

Freezing severity

1. How frequently do you experience freezing episodes?

  0 Less than once a week
  1 Not often, about once a week
  2 Often, about once a day
  3 Very often, more than once a day

2. How frequently do you experience freezing episodes during turning?

  0 Never
  1 Rarely, about once a month
  2 Not often, about once a week
  3 Often, about once a day
  4 Very often, more than once a day

3. How long is your longest freezing episode during turning?

  0 Very short, 1 second
  1 Short, 2–5 seconds
  2 Long, between 5 and 30 seconds
  3 Very long, unable to walk for more than 30 seconds

If the answer is 1 or more, go to Question 4. If the answer is 0, go directly to Question 5.

4. How frequently do you experience episodes of freezing when initiating the first step?

  0 Never
  1 Rarely, about once a month
  2 Not often, about once a week
  3 Often, about once a day
  4 Very often, more than once a day

If the answer is 1 or more go to Question 6. If the answer is 0, go directly to Question 7.

5. How long is your longest freezing episode when initiating the first step?

  0 Very short, 1 second
  1 Short, 2–5 seconds
  2 Long, between 5 and 30 seconds
  3 Very long, unable to walk for more than 30 seconds.

Freezing impact on daily life

6. How disturbing are the freezing episodes for your daily walking?

  0 Not at all
  1 Very little
  2 Moderately
  3 Significantly

7. Do the freezing episodes cause feelings of insecurity and fear of falling?

  0 Not at all
  1 Very little
  2 Moderately
  3 Significantly

8. Are your freezing episodes affecting your daily activities?

(Rate the impact of freezing on daily activities only. Not the impact of the disease in general)

  0 Not at all, I continue doing things as normal
  1 Mildly, I avoid only a few daily activities
  2 Moderately, I avoid a significant amount (about half) of daily activities
  3 Severely, I am very restricted in carrying out most daily activities.

Reprinted with the permission of the authors.

Postural Assessment Scale for Stroke (PASS)

Maintaining a posture

1. Sitting without support (sitting on the edge of a 50-cm-high examination table – a Bobath plane, for instance – with the feet touching the floor):
  0 Cannot sit
  1 Can sit with slight support, e.g. by 1 hand
  2 Can sit for more than 10 seconds without support
  3 Can sit for 5 minutes without support
2. Standing with support (feet position free, no other constraints):
  0 Cannot stand, even with support
  1 Can stand with strong support of 2 people
  2 Can stand with moderate support of 1 person
  3 Can stand with support of only 1 hand
3. Standing without support (feet position free, no other constraints):
  0 Cannot stand without support

  1 Can stand without support for 10 seconds or leans heavily on 1 leg
  2 Can stand without support for 1 minute or stands slightly asymmetrically
  3 Can stand without support for more than 1 minute and at the same time perform arm movements above the shoulder level
4. Standing on non-paretic leg (no other constraints):
  0 Cannot stand on non-paretic leg
  1 Can stand on non-paretic leg for a few seconds
  2 Can stand on non-paretic leg for more than 5 seconds
  3 Can stand on non-paretic leg for more than 10 seconds
5. Standing on paretic leg (no other constraints):
Same scoring as item 4.

Changing posture

Scoring of items 6–12 is as follows (items 6–11 are to be performed with a 50-cm-high examination table; items 10–12 are to be performed without any support; no other constraints):
  0 Cannot perform the activity
  1 Can perform the activity with much help
  2 Can perform the activity with little help
  3 Can perform the activity without help

6. Supine to affected side lateral
7. Supine to non-affected side lateral
8. Supine to sitting up on the edge of the table
9. Sitting on the edge of the table to supine
10. Sitting to standing up
11. Standing up to sitting down
12. Standing, picking up a pencil from the floor

PASS-3 Level

The 5-item PASS-3L contains the same five items as the 'Maintaining a posture' section of the original PASS. However, scoring criteria consists of only three levels: 0, 1.5 and 3. Scoring criteria is as follows:

Scoring criteria:

Items 1–4:

0   Cannot perform the activity
1.5   Can perform the activity with help
3   Can perform the activity without help.

Item 5:

0   Cannot stand on non-paretic leg for a few seconds
1.5   Can stand on non-paretic leg for a few seconds (but less than 10 seconds)
3   Can stand on non-paretic leg for more than 10 seconds.

Reproduced from Benaim C, Pérennou A, Villy J, Rousseaux M, Yvon Pelissier J 1999 Validation of a Standardized Assessment of Postural Control in Stroke Patients. Stroke 1999 30:1862-1868, with permission from Wolters Kluwer Health.

Short Parkinson's Evaluation Scale (SPES/SCOPA)

Motor evaluation

Clinical examination

Rest tremor

Assess each arm separately during 20 seconds; hands rest on thighs; if tremor is not evident at rest, try to keep the patient attentive, e.g. by having them count backwards with eyes closed.

0 Absent
1 Small amplitude (<1 cm) occurring spontaneously, or obtained only while keeping patient attentive (any amplitude)
2 Moderate amplitude (1–4 cm), occurring spontaneously
3 Large amplitude (≥4 cm), occurring spontaneously.

Postural tremor

Check with arms outstretched, pronated and semi-pronated, and with index fingers of both hands almost touching each other (elbows flexed); assess each position during 20 seconds.

0 Absent
1 Small amplitude (<1 cm)
2 Moderate amplitude (1–4 cm)
3 Large amplitude (≥4 cm).

Rapid alternating movements of hands

Rapid alternating pronation/supination movements of upper hand, each time slapping the palm of the horizontally held lower hand during 20 seconds; each hand separately.

0 Normal
1 Slow execution, or mild slowing and/or reduction in amplitude; may have occasional arrests
2 Moderate slowing and/or reduction in amplitude or hesitations in initiating movements or frequent arrests in ongoing movements
3 Can barely perform task.

Rigidity

Assess passive movements of elbow and wrist over full range, with the patient relaxed in sitting position; ignore cogwheeling; check each arm separately.

0 Absent
1 Mild rigidity over full range, no difficulty reaching end-positions
2 Moderate rigidity, some difficulties reaching end-positions
3 Severe rigidity, considerable difficulties reaching end-positions.

Rise from chair

Patient is instructed to fold arms across chest; use straight back chair.

0 Normal
1 Slowly; does not need arms to get up
2 Needs arms to get up (can get up without help)
3 Unable to rise (without help).

Postural stability

Stand behind the patient and pull patient backwards, while patient is standing erect with eyes open and feet spaced slightly apart; patient is *not* prepared.

0 Normal, may take up to two steps to recover
1 Takes three or more steps; recovers unaided
2 Would fall if not caught
3 Spontaneous tendency to fall or unable to stand unaided.

Gait

Assess gait pattern; use walking aid or offer assistance, if necessary.

0 Normal
1 Mild slowing and/or reduction of step height or length; does not shuffle
2 Severe slowing, or shuffles, or has festination
3 Unable to walk.

Speech

0 Normal
1 Slight loss of expression, diction, and/or volume
2 Slurred; not always intelligible
3 Unintelligible always or most of the time.

Historical information

Freezing during 'on'

Freezing is characterized by hesitation when trying to start walking or being 'glued' to the ground while walking.

0 Absent
1 Start hesitation only, occasionally present
2 Frequently present, may have freezing when walking
3 Severe freezing when walking.

Activities of daily living

Speech

0 Normal
1 Some difficulty; may sometimes be asked to repeat sentences
2 Considerable difficulty; frequently asked to repeat sentences
3 Unintelligible most of the time.

Feeding (cutting, filling cup, etc.)

0 Normal
1 Some difficulty or slow; does not need assistance
2 Considerable difficulty; may need some assistance
3 Needs almost complete or complete assistance.

Dressing

0 Normal
1 Some difficulty or slow; does not need assistance
2 Considerable difficulty; may need some assistance—for instance, buttoning, getting arms into sleeves
3 Needs almost complete or complete assistance.

Hygiene (washing, combing hair, shaving, brushing teeth, using toilet)

0 Normal
1 Some difficulty or slow; does not need assistance
2 Considerable difficulty; may need some assistance
3 Needs almost complete or complete assistance.

Swallowing

0 Normal
1 Some difficulty or slow; does not choke; normal diet
2 Sometimes chokes; may require soft food
3 Chokes frequently; may require soft food or alternative method of food intake.

Changing position (turning over in bed, getting up out of bed, getting up out of a chair, turning around when standing)

0 Normal
1 Some difficulty or slow; does not need assistance with any change of position
2 Considerable difficulty; may need assistance with one or more changes of position
3 Needs almost complete or complete assistance with one or more changes of position.

Walking

0 Normal
1 Some difficulty or slow; does not need assistance or walking aid
2 Considerable difficulty; may need assistance or walking aid
3 Unable to walk, or walks only with assistance and great effort.

Handwriting

0 Normal
1 Some difficulty, for instance, slow, small letters; all words legible
2 Considerable difficulty; not all words legible; may need to use block letters
3 Majority of words are illegible.

Motor complications

Dyskinesias (presence)

0 Absent
1 Present some of the time
2 Present a considerable part of the time
3 Present most or all of the time.

Dyskinesias (severity)

0 Absent
1 Small amplitude
2 Moderate amplitude
3 Large amplitude.

Motor fluctuations (presence of 'off' periods)

What proportion of the waking day is patient 'off' on average?

0 None
1 Some of the time
2 A considerable part of the time
3 Most or all of the time.

Motor fluctuations (severity of 'off' periods)

0 Absent
1 Mild end-of-dose fluctuations
2 Moderate end-of-dose fluctuations; unpredictable fluctuations may occur occasionally
3 Severe end-of-dose fluctuations; unpredictable on–off oscillations occur frequently.

Reproduced from Marinus J, Visser M, Stiggelbout A M, Rabey J M, Martinez-Martin P, Bonuccelli U, Kraus P H, van Hilten J J. A short scale for the assessment of motor impairments and disabilities in Parkinson's disease: the SPES/SCOPA. Journal of neurology, neurosurgery, and psychiatry 2004 75:388-395, with permission from BMJ Publishing Group

Motor Assessment Scale (MAS)

If the patient cannot complete any part of a section, score a zero (0) for that section. There are nine sections in all.

Supine to side-lying onto intact side (starting position: supine with knees straight)

1. Uses intact arm to pull body toward intact side. Uses intact leg to hook impaired leg to pull it over.
2. Actively moves impaired leg across body to roll but leaves impaired arm behind.
3. Impaired arm is lifted across body with other arm. Impaired leg moves actively and body follows as a block.
4. Actively moves impaired arm across body. The rest of the body moves as a block.
5. Actively moves impaired arm and leg rolling to intact side but overbalances.
6. Rolls to intact side in 3 seconds without use of hands.

Score: _____

Supine to sitting over side of bed

1. Patient assisted to the side-lying position: patient lifts head sideways but cannot sit up.
2. Patient may be assisted to side-lying and is assisted to sitting but has head control throughout.
3. Patient may be assisted to side-lying and is assisted with lowering lower extremities (LEs) off bed to assume sitting.
4. Patient may be assisted to side-lying but is able to sit up without help.
5. Patient able to move from supine to sitting without help.
6. Patient able to move from supine to sitting without help in 10 seconds.

Score: _____

Balance sitting

1. Patient is assisted to sitting and needs support to remain sitting.
2. Patient sits unsupported for 10 seconds with arms folded, knees and feet together, with feet on the floor.
3. Patient sits unsupported with weight shifted forwards and evenly distributed over both hips/legs. Head and thoracic spine extended.
4. Patient sits unsupported with feet together on the floor, hands resting on thighs. Without moving the legs, the patient turns the head and trunk to look behind the right and left shoulders.
5. Patient sits unsupported with feet together on the floor. Without allowing the legs or feet to move and without holding on, the patient must reach forward to touch the floor (10 cm or 4 inches in front of them). The affected arm may be supported if necessary.
6. Patient sits on a stool unsupported with feet on the floor. Patient reaches sideways without moving the legs or holding on and returns to sitting position. Support affected arm if needed.

Score: _____

Sitting to standing

1. Patient assisted to standing – any method.
2. Patient assisted to standing. The patient's weight is unevenly distributed and may use hands for support.
3. Patient stands up. The patient's weight is evenly distributed but hips and knees are flexed – no use of hands for support.
4. Patient stands up. Remains standing for 5 seconds with hips and knees extended with weight evenly distributed.
5. Patient stands up and sits down again. When standing, hips and knees are extended with weight evenly distributed.
6. Patient stands up and sits down again 3 times in 10 seconds, with hips and knees extended and weight evenly distributed.

Score: _____

Walking

1. With assistance, the patient stands on affected leg with the affected weight-bearing hip extended, and steps forward with the intact leg.
2. Walks with the assistance of one person.
3. Walks 10 feet or 3 metres without assistance but with an assistive device.

4. Walks 16 feet or 5 metres without a device or assistance in 15 seconds.

5. Walks 33 feet or 10 metres without assistance or a device. Is able to pick up a small object from the floor with either hand and walk back in 25 seconds.

6. Walks up and down 4 steps with or without a device but without holding on to a rail 3 times in 35 seconds.

Score: _____

General tonus (tick one – add '6' to score if tone on affected side is normal)

1. Flaccid, limp, no resistance when body parts are handled.

2. Some resistance felt as body parts are moved.

3. Variable, sometimes flaccid, sometimes good tone, sometimes hypertonic.

7. Hypertonic 50% of the time

5. Hypertonic all of the time

6. Consistently normal response

Score: _____

This test is designed to assess the return of function following a stroke or other neurological impairment. The test looks at a patient's ability to move with low tone or in a synergistic pattern and finally move actively out of that pattern into normal movement.

The higher the score, the higher functioning the patient is on the affected side.

- High score: 54
- Low score: 0.

Reproduced from Carr JH, Shepherd RB, Nordholm L, Lynne D. Investigation of a New Motor Assessment Scale for Stroke Patients. Physical Therapy 1985 65(2), with permission of the American Physical Therapy Association. This material is copyrighted, and any further reproduction or distribution is prohibited.

Upper-limb items on the MAS (proposed by Sabrai et al 2005)

Upper-arm function

1. Lying, protract shoulder girdle with arm in elevation. (Therapist places arm in position and supports it with elbow in extension.)

2. Lying, hold extended arm in elevation for 2 seconds. (Therapist should place arm in position and patient must maintain position with some external rotation. Elbow must be held within 20° of full extension.)

3. Flexion and extension of elbow to take palm to forehead with arm as in 2. (Therapist may assist supination of forearm.)

4. Sitting, hold extended arm in forward flexion at 90° to body for 2 seconds. (Therapist should place arm in position and patient must maintain position with some external rotation and elbow extension. Do not allow excess shoulder elevation.)

5. Sitting, patient lifts arm to above position, holds it there for 10 seconds, and then lowers it. (Patient must maintain position with some external rotation. Do not allow pronation.)

6. Standing, hand against wall. Maintain arm position while turning body towards wall. (Have arm abducted to 90° with palm flat against the wall.)

Hand movements

1. Sitting, extension of wrist. (Therapist should have patient sitting at a table with forearm resting on the table. Therapist places cylindrical object in palm of patient's hand. Patient is asked to lift object off the table by extending the wrist. Do not allow elbow flexion.)

2. Sitting, radial deviation of wrist. (Therapist should place forearm in mid-pronation-supination, i.e. resting on the ulnar side, thumb in line with the forearm and wrist in extension, fingers around a cylindrical object. Patient is asked to lift hand off table. Do not allow elbow flexion or pronation.)

3. Sitting, elbow into side, pronation and supination. (Elbow unsupported and at a right angle. Three-quarter range is acceptable.)

4. Reach forward, pick up large ball of 14-cm (5-in) diameter with both hands and put it down. (Ball should be on table so far in front of patient that he has to extend arms fully to reach it. Shoulders must be protracted, elbow extended, wrist neutral or extended. Palms should be kept in contact with the ball.)

5. Pick up a polystyrene cup from the table and put it on the table across the other side of the body. (Do not allow alteration in shape of the cup.)

6. Continuous opposition of thumb and each finger more than 14 times in 10 seconds. (Each finger in turn taps the thumb, starting with index finger. Do not allow thumb to slide from one finger to the other, or to go backwards.)

Advanced hand activities

1. Picking up the top of a pen and putting it down again. (Patient stretches arm forward, picks up pen top, releases it on to table close to body.)
2. Picking up 1 jellybean from a cup and placing it in another cup. (Teacup contains eight jellybeans. Both cups must be at arms' length. Left hand takes jellybean from cup on right and releases it in cup on left.)
3. Drawing horizontal lines to stop at a vertical line 10 times in 20 seconds. (At least 5 lines must touch and stop at the vertical line.)
4. Holding a pencil, making rapid consecutive dots on a sheet of paper. (Patient must do at least 2 dots a second for 5 seconds. Patient picks pencil up and positions it without assistance. Patient must hold pen as for writing. Patient must make a dot not a stroke.)
5. Taking a dessert spoon of liquid to the mouth. (Do not allow head to lower towards spoon. Do not allow liquid to spill.)
6. Holding a comb and combing hair at back of head.

Appendix 5: Patient satisfaction

Introduction

This Appendix contains the outcome measures discussed in Chapter 11. In Tables 11.1 and 11.2 (in Ch. 11) there are listed links to a website where an electronic copy of the outcome variable is available.

This Appendix contains the following patient satisfaction surveys:

- Physical Therapy Outpatient Satisfaction Survey (POPTS)
- European POPTS
- Chest Physiotherapy Satisfaction Survey
- Physical Therapy Patient Satisfaction Questionnaire
- MedRisk
- Physiotherapy outpatients satisfaction questionnaire
- Patient Satisfaction Questionnaire.

DOI: 10.1016/B978-0-443-06915-4.00016-4

Physical Therapy Outpatient Satisfaction Survey (PTOPS)

Administration

5-point Likert scale: 1 = Strongly disagree; 2 = Disagree; 3 = Uncertain; 4 = Agree; 5 = Strongly agree.

Administration time = approximately 6–10 minutes. Items to be re-coded: 9, 10, 16, 17, 19, 21, 25, 28, 30 (1 = 5, 2 = 4, 4 = 2, 5 = 1)

1. The cost of treatment is more than I expected
2. I enjoy listening to my therapist
3. I expect the facility to be quieter than it is
4. The facility is flexible about payment options
5. The distance required to get to the facility is acceptable to me
6. I expect my therapist to spend more time with me than he/she does
7. I am given privacy when I need it
8. It is difficult for me to get into the facility from the parking lot
9. I am charged a reasonable amount for my therapy
10. This facility could be more conveniently located for me
11. I feel my therapist overcharges me
12. The office staff is attentive to my needs
13. My therapist acts like he/she is doing me a big favour by treating me
14. The facility is in a desirable location
15. My therapist could communicate with me more
16. I have to wait too long between appointments
17. The quality of the care I receive is not compatible with the cost
18. This facility is a nice place to get my therapy
19. It is somewhat difficult for me to reach this PT facility
20. The facility is too crowded
21. I have to travel too far to receive my treatment
22. I can get around easily inside of the facility
23. I don't really enjoy talking with my therapist
24. My therapist seems to have a genuine interest in me as a person
25. My therapist does not expect me to pay significantly more than what my insurance covers
26. I anticipate my questions will be answered clearly
27. My therapist doesn't give me a chance to say what is on my mind
28. I should not have to travel this far for therapy
29. This facility appreciates my business
30. It could be easier to make the arrangements to pay for my therapy
31. My therapist should be more thorough in my treatment
32. The physical therapy facility is conveniently located for me
33. My therapist should listen more carefully to what I tell him/her
34. I get along well with everyone in this PT facility

Mean subscale scores (four separate scores):

- Enhancers: 2, 7, 12, 16, 18, 22, 24, 26, 29, 34.
- Location: 5, 10, 14, 19, 21, 28, 32.
- Detractors: 3, 6, 8, 13, 15, 20, 23, 27, 31, 33.
- Cost: 1, 4, 9, 11, 17, 25, 30.

Interpretation

Enhancers and Location are positive scales, i.e. higher scores indicate greater satisfaction. Detractors and Cost are negative scales, i.e. higher scores indicate less satisfaction.

European POPTS

Section (i)

Please answer the following questions regarding your overall satisfaction with your physiotherapy treatment. Mark an X next to the ONE answer that most closely agrees with your personal opinions regarding your experience.

1. What are the chances that you would recommend this physiotherapy clinic to family or friends?

☐ Poor

☐ Fair

☐ Good

☐ Very good

☐ Excellent

2. How would you rate your overall satisfaction with your experience at this physiotherapy clinic?

☐ Poor

☐ Fair

☐ Good

☐ Very good

☐ Excellent

3. If you needed physiotherapy again, what are the chances that you would return to this physiotherapy clinic?

☐ Poor

☐ Fair

☐ Good

☐ Very good

☐ Excellent

Section (ii)

Please answer the following questions regarding specific details of your physiotherapy experience at this physiotherapy clinic. Mark an X next to the single answer that most closely agrees with your personal opinions.

4. The cost of treatment was more than I expected.

☐ Strongly disagree

☐ Disagree

☐ Neither agree nor disagree

☐ Agree

☐ Strongly agree

5. I enjoyed listening to my physiotherapist.

☐ Strongly disagree

☐ Disagree

☐ Neither agree nor disagree

☐ Agree

☐ Strongly agree

6. I expected the physiotherapy clinic to be quieter than it was.

☐ Strongly disagree

☐ Disagree

☐ Neither agree nor disagree

☐ Agree

☐ Strongly agree

7. The physiotherapy clinic was flexible about payment options.

☐ Strongly disagree

☐ Disagree

☐ Neither agree nor disagree

☐ Agree

☐ Strongly agree

8. The distance required to get to the physiotherapy clinic was acceptable to me.

   ☐ Strongly disagree

   ☐ Disagree

   ☐ Neither agree nor disagree

   ☐ Agree

   ☐ Strongly agree

9. I expected my physiotherapist to spend more time with me than he/she did.

   ☐ Strongly disagree

   ☐ Disagree

   ☐ Neither agree nor disagree

   ☐ Agree

   ☐ Strongly agree

10. I was given privacy when I needed it.

    ☐ Strongly disagree

    ☐ Disagree

    ☐ Neither agree nor disagree

    ☐ Agree

    ☐ Strongly agree

11. It was difficult for me to get into the physiotherapy clinic from the car park.

    ☐ Strongly disagree

    ☐ Disagree

    ☐ Neither agree nor disagree

    ☐ Agree

    ☐ Strongly agree

12. I was charged a reasonable amount for my physiotherapy.

    ☐ Strongly disagree

    ☐ Disagree

    ☐ Neither agree nor disagree

    ☐ Agree

    ☐ Strongly agree

13. This physiotherapy clinic could have been more conveniently located for me.

    ☐ Strongly disagree

    ☐ Disagree

    ☐ Neither agree nor disagree

    ☐ Agree

    ☐ Strongly agree

14. I felt my physiotherapist overcharged me.

    ☐ Strongly disagree

    ☐ Disagree

    ☐ Neither agree nor disagree

    ☐ Agree

    ☐ Strongly agree

15. The office staff were attentive to my needs.

    ☐ Strongly disagree

    ☐ Disagree

    ☐ Neither agree nor disagree

    ☐ Agree

    ☐ Strongly agree

16. My physiotherapist acted like he/she was doing a big favour by treating me.

    ☐ Strongly disagree

    ☐ Disagree

    ☐ Neither agree nor disagree

    ☐ Agree

    ☐ Strongly agree

17. The physiotherapy clinic was in a desirable location

    ☐ Strongly disagree

    ☐ Disagree

    ☐ Neither agree nor disagree

    ☐ Agree

    ☐ Strongly agree

18. My physiotherapist could have communicated with me more.

☐ Strongly disagree

☐ Disagree

☐ Neither agree nor disagree

☐ Agree

☐ Strongly agree

19. I had to wait too long between appointments.

☐ Strongly disagree

☐ Disagree

☐ Neither agree nor disagree

☐ Agree

☐ Strongly agree

20. The quality of the care I received was NOT compatible with the cost.

☐ Strongly disagree

☐ Disagree

☐ Neither agree nor disagree

☐ Agree

☐ Strongly agree

21. This physiotherapy clinic was a nice place to get my physiotherapy.

☐ Strongly disagree

☐ Disagree

☐ Neither agree nor disagree

☐ Agree

☐ Strongly agree

22. It was somewhat difficult for me to reach this physiotherapy clinic.

☐ Strongly disagree

☐ Disagree

☐ Neither agree nor disagree

☐ Agree

☐ Strongly agree

23. The physiotherapy clinic was too crowded.

☐ Strongly disagree

☐ Disagree

☐ Neither agree nor disagree

☐ Agree

☐ Strongly agree

24. I had to travel too far to receive my treatment.

☐ Strongly disagree

☐ Disagree

☐ Neither agree nor disagree

☐ Agree

☐ Strongly agree

25. I could get around easily inside of the physiotherapy clinic.

☐ Strongly disagree

☐ Disagree

☐ Neither agree nor disagree

☐ Agree

☐ Strongly agree

26. I didn't really enjoy talking with my physiotherapist.

☐ Strongly disagree

☐ Disagree

☐ Neither agree nor disagree

☐ Agree

☐ Strongly agree

27. My physiotherapist seemed to have a genuine interest in me as a person.

☐ Strongly disagree

☐ Disagree

☐ Neither agree nor disagree

☐ Agree

☐ Strongly agree

28. My physiotherapist did not expect me to pay significantly more than my insurance covered.

☐ Strongly disagree

☐ Disagree

☐ Neither agree nor disagree

☐ Agree

☐ Strongly agree

29. I anticipated my questions would be answered clearly.

☐ Strongly disagree

☐ Disagree

☐ Neither agree nor disagree

☐ Agree

☐ Strongly agree

30. My physiotherapist didn't give me a chance to say what was on my mind.

☐ Strongly disagree

☐ Disagree

☐ Neither agree nor disagree

☐ Agree

☐ Strongly agree

31. I should not have had to travel this far for physiotherapy.

☐ Strongly disagree

☐ Disagree

☐ Neither agree nor disagree

☐ Agree

☐ Strongly agree

32. This physiotherapy clinic appreciated my business.

☐ Strongly disagree

☐ Disagree

☐ Neither agree nor disagree

☐ Agree

☐ Strongly agree

33. It could have been easier to make the arrangements to pay for my physiotherapy.

☐ Strongly disagree

☐ Disagree

☐ Neither agree nor disagree

☐ Agree

☐ Strongly agree

34. My physiotherapist should have been more thorough in my treatment.

☐ Strongly disagree

☐ Disagree

☐ Neither agree nor disagree

☐ Agree

☐ Strongly agree

35. The physiotherapy clinic was conveniently located for me.

☐ Strongly disagree

☐ Disagree

☐ Neither agree nor disagree

☐ Agree

☐ Strongly agree

36. My physiotherapist should have listened more carefully to what I told him/her.

☐ Strongly disagree

☐ Disagree

☐ Neither agree nor disagree

☐ Agree

☐ Strongly agree

37. I got along well with everyone in this physiotherapy clinic.

☐ Strongly disagree

☐ Disagree

☐ Neither agree nor disagree

☐ Agree

☐ Strongly agree

Section (iii)

We need to study the relationship between your treatment and how satisfied you are. Please answer the following questions regarding your treatment by marking an X in the box beside the correct answer.

38. How would you rate the improvement in your condition as a result of your physiotherapy treatment?

☐ Poor

☐ Fair

☐ Good

☐ Very good

☐ Excellent

39. What type of injury or illness caused you to seek treatment at this physiotherapy clinic? (Choose the main problem area)

☐ Neck problem

☐ Back problem

☐ Shoulder problem

☐ Elbow problem

☐ Wrist/hand problem

☐ Hip problem

☐ Knee problem

☐ Ankle/foot problem

☐ Other (please specify) _____

_____

40. What type of treatment did you receive? *(Mark all that apply)*

☐ Advice and information (e.g. posture, weight management, back care education, etc.)

☐ Manual physiotherapy (e.g. manual traction, massage, joint mobilization or manipulation)

☐ Use of devices and equipment (e.g. sticks, braces, crutches, orthotics, etc.)

☐ Cardiovascular exercises (e.g. walking, swimming, cycling, etc.)

☐ Exercise therapy (e.g. stretching or strengthening exercises, core exercises, resistance exercises, etc.)

☐ Electrotherapy treatment (e.g. Ultrasound, laser, interferential, heat or ice therapy)

☐ Group exercise or therapy classes

☐ Home exercise programme

☐ Other (please specify) _____

_____

_____

41. Was this your first experience with physiotherapy?

☐ Yes

☐ No

42. How did you arrange to pay for this episode of physiotherapy treatment? (Choose the major source)

☐ Self-funded

☐ VHI

☐ BUPA

☐ Work insurance scheme

☐ Other (please specify) _____

43. What was the total cost of the treatment? (Estimate if unsure)

€ _____

44. Roughly, how many times did you attend the physiotherapy clinic?

(Indicate if this is an approximate number)

_____

Section (iv)

Finally, we would like to understand how personal characteristics influence patient satisfaction. Please answer the following questions about yourself. Mark the correct box, or fill in the blank, as appropriate.

45. What is your sex or gender? (Choose one)

☐ Male

☐ Female

46. What is your race/ethnicity?

☐ Black

☐ White

☐ Asian

☐ Hispanic

☐ Indian

☐ Other (please specify) _____

47. What is your marital status?

☐ Married

☐ Living together as married

☐ Divorced

☐ Widowed

☐ Separated

☐ Never married

☐ Other (please specify) _____

48. What is your age?

☐ 18–20

☐ 21–25

☐ 26–30

☐ 31–35

☐ 36–40

☐ 41–45

☐ 46–50

☐ 51–55

☐ 56–60

☐ 61–65

49. What is the highest year in secondary school you have completed?

☐ Did not attend secondary school

☐ 1st Year

☐ 2nd year

☐ 3rd year

☐ 4th year

☐ 5th year

☐ 6th year

50. Do you have a degree or other professional qualification?

☐ Yes

☐ No

If yes please specify _____

51. What is your current employment status?

☐ Employed/working for payment or profit

☐ Looking for first regular job

☐ Unemployed

☐ Student

☐ Looking after home/family

☐ Retired from employment

☐ Unable to work due to sickness or disability

52. What is your normal main occupation?

_____

53. What was the name of the Physiotherapy Clinic which you attended?

(if you wish to include this information)

_____

If you have feedback (positive or negative) regarding this questionnaire, your comments would be very helpful and greatly appreciated.

If you have any other feedback (positive or negative) regarding the physiotherapist and the physiotherapy clinics, your comments would be very helpful and greatly appreciated.

Reprinted with the permission of the author.

Chest Physiotherapy Satisfaction Survey©

Patient Number: _____ Date: _____

Therapy type: _____

Please answer the following questions by circling a number from 1 to 5. Circle **1** if you *Strongly disagree* with the statement through to **5** if you *Strongly agree* with the statement.

	Strongly agree		⟷		**Strongly disagree**
This type of chest PT helps me/my child cough up mucus	1	2	3	4	5
This type of chest PT helps me/my child breathe better	1	2	3	4	5
This type of chest PT helps during illness or infection	1	2	3	4	5
This type of chest PT helps to maintain lung function over time	1	2	3	4	5
Overall, this type of chest PT is effective	1	2	3	4	5
This type of chest PT is simple to do	1	2	3	4	5
This type of chest PT can be done anywhere	1	2	3	4	5
This type of chest PT is easy to fit into our daily schedule	1	2	3	4	5
This type of chest PT allows better use of my/my child's time	1	2	3	4	5
Overall, this type of chest PT is convenient	1	2	3	4	5
This type of chest PT causes chest pain or discomfort	1	2	3	4	5
This type of chest PT causes excessive coughing spells	1	2	3	4	5
This type of chest PT causes difficulty breathing	1	2	3	4	5
This type of chest PT causes other physical problems	1	2	3	4	5
Overall, this type of chest PT is well tolerated	1	2	3	4	5
I am satisfied with this type of chest PT	1	2	3	4	5
I would like to continue with this type of chest PT	1	2	3	4	5

Physical Therapy Patient Satisfaction Questionnaire

Dear Patient

You recently received physical therapy services at our facility. Because we strive to deliver the best possible physical therapy service, we are interested in learning from patients how we might improve or enhance our services. Please take a few moments to complete and return this questionnaire.

Please place an X in the appropriate box to indicate your rating, or answer the descriptive questions on the appropriate line. Any additional comments you wish to make are welcome; write in the 'Comments' sections at the end of the questionnaire, or attach additional pages if you require more space. Please return the questionnaire to us at your earliest convenience.

Thank you very much for your feedback!

Descriptive Questions

1. Your age: _____ (years)

2. Your sex: ☐ Male; ☐ Female

3. How did you learn about this facility? (Tick all that apply.)

☐ Physician

☐ Insurance company recommendation

☐ Friend

☐ Former patient

☐ Telephone book

☐ Other, please indicate _____

4. Was this your first experience with physical therapy?

Yes ☐   No ☐

5. Was this your first experience with this facility?

Yes ☐   No ☐

6. Please check the location of the problem for which you received physical therapy. (Check all that apply).

☐ Neck

☐ Hip

☐ Lower back

☐ Foot

☐ Shoulder

☐ Hand

☐ Elbow

☐ Knee

☐ Other, please indicate _____

Please rate your degree of satisfaction with each of the following statements. 1 = strongly disagree, 2 = disagree, 3 = neither agree nor disagree, 4 = agree, 5 = strongly agree. Please tick (9) if you have No opinion on the subject.

	Strongly disagree (1)	Disagree (2)	Neither agree nor disagree (3)	Agree (4)	Strongly agree (5)	No opinion (9)
7. My privacy was respected during my physical therapy care.						
8. My physical therapist courteous.						

Continued

181

	Strongly disagree (1)	Disagree (2)	Neither agree nor disagree (3)	Agree (4)	Strongly agree (5)	No opinion (9)
9. All other staff members were courteous.						
10. The clinic scheduled appointments at convenient times.						
11. I was satisfied with the treatment provided by my physical therapist.						
12. My first visit for physical therapy was scheduled quickly.						
13. It was easy to schedule visits after my appointment.						
14. I was seen promptly when I arrived for treatment.						
15. The location of the facility was convenient for me.						
16. My bills were accurate.						
17. I was satisfied with the services provided by my physical therapist assistant(s).						
18. Parking was available for me.						
19. My physical therapist understood my problem or condition.						
20. The instructions my physical therapist gave me were helpful.						
21. I was satisfied with the overall quality of my physical therapy care.						
22. I would recommend this facility to family or friends.						
23. I would return to this facility if I required physical therapy care in the future.						
24. The cost of the physical therapy treatment received was reasonable.						
25. If I had to, I would pay for these physical therapy services myself.						
26. Overall, I was satisfied with my experience with physical therapy.						

Comments:

_____

_____

_____

_____

MedRisk

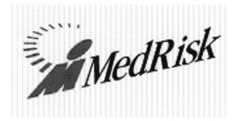

Patient survey

Please answer the following questions:

1. Age: _____ (years)

2. Male ☐; Female ☐

3. General area of treatment (tick all that apply)

- ☐   Neck
- ☐   Back
- ☐   Arm
- ☐   Leg
- ☐   Foot/ankle
- ☐   Hand/wrist
- ☐   Other (specify) _____

4. Did you complete your course of treatment?

- ☐ Yes
- ☐ No: Date of last treatment: _____

5. Have you returned to work?

- ☐   No
- ☐   Yes: Date returned to work: _____
- ☐   Not applicable/did not work prior to injury
- ☐   Injury did not keep me out of work

6. How were you injured?

- ☐ On the job
- ☐ Personal injury
- ☐ Other _____

In the recent past you received Physical Therapy for your condition. We are interested in understanding your thoughts about the treatment you received.

Please answer the questions below by circling the response which best describes your opinions about your Physical Therapy treatment.

		Strongly disagree	Disagree	Neutral	Agree	Strongly agree
1.	The office receptionist is courteous.	1	2	3	4	5
2.	The registration process is appropriate.	1	2	3	4	5
3.	The waiting area is comfortable.	1	2	3	4	5
4.	My therapist does not spend enough time with me.	1	2	3	4	5
5.	My therapist thoroughly explains the treatment(s) I receive.	1	2	3	4	5
6.	My therapist treats me respectfully.	1	2	3	4	5
7.	My therapist does not listen to my concerns.	1	2	3	4	5

Continued

	Strongly disagree	Disagree	Neutral	Agree	Strongly agree
8. My therapist answers all my questions.	1	2	3	4	5
9. My therapist advises me on ways to avoid future problems.	1	2	3	4	5
10. My therapist gives me detailed instructions regarding my home programme.	1	2	3	4	5
11. Overall, I am completely satisfied with the service I receive from my therapist.	1	2	3	4	5
12. I would return to this office for future services or care.	1	2	3	4	5

13. How does your current condition compare to how it was before you started physical therapy treatment? (Circle comment that best fits)

1	2	3	4	5	6	7	8	9
Very much better	Much better	Somewhat better	Slightly better	Same	Slightly worse	Somewhat worse	Much worse	Very much worse

Below you may briefly comment on any area of your treatment that was not addressed by the questions above.

_____

_____

_____

_____

Reprinted with the permission of the author.

Physiotherapy Outpatients Satisfaction Questionnaire

1. My therapist gave me confidence that I was going to get better.
2. I was not always seen promptly for my treatment sessions.
3. I did not have confidence that the therapist knew what (s)he was doing.
4. I should have got a better result from the treatment I was given in this department.
5. I expected the treatment would help relieve my pain.
6. My therapist did not listen to what I had to say.
7. I have made a full recovery as a result of treatment.
8. I did not have any of my treatment sessions cancelled.
9. I expected the treatment would get me better.
10. The treatment helped me at the time but the effect did not last.
11. My therapist gave me encouragement and praise.
12. I was not happy to be left to work on my own during the session.
13. I expected the treatment would cure my problem.
14. The treatment was too rushed.
15. I am completely satisfied with all aspects of my visits to the physiotherapy department.
16. The therapist explained my condition to me in great detail.
17. I did not think treatment would be able to help me.
18. I was able to choose the appointment times for my treatment.
19. The treatment has helped me in some way but I am not completely better.
20. My therapist did not seem interested in me.
21. It was important for me to see the same therapist throughout my treatment.
22. The treatment was tailored to my needs.
23. I was able to ask the therapist about anything connected with my treatment.
24. I had to wait a long time to get my first appointment for treatment.
25. The treatment sessions were too short.
26. The treatment has not helped me at all.
27. My therapist put me at ease and was very kind to me.
28. The therapist did not answer all my questions.
29. I got on very well with my therapist.
30. Treatment sessions were too infrequent to get any benefit.
31. I am now completely pain free as a result of treatment.
32. I was made aware of my responsibilities in managing my condition as a result of treatment.
33. I did not have the undivided attention of the therapist during my treatment.
34. I am completely satisfied with the treatment I received in this department.
35. I have regained full mobility as a result of treatment.
36. I was able to contact the department for help if I had any further problems after discharge.
37. The quality of service I received in this department could have been better.
38. The treatment was fully explained to me.

Note: Item statements are presented in the order in which they appear in the questionnaire. However, the style of the questionnaire is not reproduced here.

Scoring:

5-point Likert scale: 5 = Strongly agree; 4 = Agree; 3 = Not sure; 2 = Disagree; 1 = Strongly disagree.

Reversed scoring items: 2, 3, 4, 6, 10, 12, 14, 17, 19, 20, 24, 25, 26, 28, 30, 33, 37 (5 = 1, 4 = 2, 2 = 4, 1 = 5).

Items in each of the six subscales: Expectations: 1, 5, 9, 13, 17; Therapist: 11, 20, 21, 27, 29, 32; Communication: 3, 6, 16, 23, 28, 38; Organization: 2, 8, 12, 14, 25, 30, 33, 36; Clinical outcome: 7, 10, 19, 26, 31, 35; Satisfaction: 4, 15, 18, 22, 24, 34, 37.

Reproduced from Hills, R. and Kitchen, S. Satisfaction with outpatient physiotherapy: Focus groups to explore the views of patients with acute and chronic musculoskeletal conditions. Physiotherapy Theory and Practice 2007 15:147-154. with permission from Informa Healthcare.

Patient Satisfaction Questionnaire

This questionnaire concerns the physical therapy you received at your hospital. Your answers will help us improve our services. Please answer each item by ticking the most appropriate box. There are no right or wrong answers. Your answers will be treated confidentially.

	Poor	Fair	Good	Very good	Excellent
Ease of administrative admission procedures					
Courtesy and helpfulness of secretary					
Simplicity of scheduling and time to get first appointment					
Ability of physical therapist to put you at ease and reassure you					
Explanations about what will be done to you during treatment					
Quality of information you received at the end of the treatment regarding the future					
Feeling of security at all times during the treatment					
Extent to which treatment was adapted to your problem					
Ease of access of physical therapy facilities					
Indications to help you find your way around and in hospital buildings					
Comfort of the room where physical therapy was provided					
Calm and relaxing atmosphere in physical therapy rooms					
Your physical therapy overall					

	Certainly not	Probably not	Not sure	Yes, probably	Yes, certainly
Would you recommend this facility to people close to you?					

Thank you for your help.

Index

Note: Page numbers followed by *b* indicate boxes, *f* indicate figures and *t* indicate tables.